How to
Feel
Fabulous
Today!

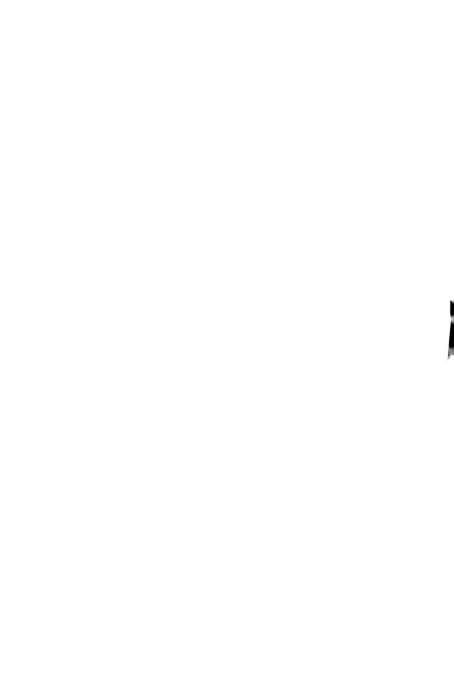

How to Feel Fabulous Today!

250 Simple and Natural Ways to Achieve Spiritual, Emotional, and Physical Well-Being

Stephanie Tourles

STOREY BOOKS

Schoolhouse Road
Pownal, Vermont 05261

*The mission of Storey Communications is to serve our customers
by publishing practical information that encourages personal independence
in harmony with the environment.*

This publication is intended to provide educational information for the reader on the covered subject. It is not intended to take the place of personalized medical counseling, diagnosis, and treatment from a trained health professional.

Edited by Deborah Balmuth and Marie Salter
Cover design by Leslie Constantino
Cover photograph/illustration by PhotoDisc/Art Explosion
Text design by Susan Bernier and Jennifer Jepson Smith
Text production by Jennifer Jepson Smith
Indexed by Gwen Steege

Printed in the United States by R.R. Donnelley
10 9 8 7 6 5 4 3 2 1

Library of Congress Cataloging-in-Publication Data

Tourles, Stephanie L., 1962–
   How to feel fabulous today!: 250 simple and natural ways to achieve
   spiritual, emotional, and physical well-being / by Stephanie Tourles.
      p.   cm.
   Includes index.
   ISBN 1-58017-313-6 (alk. paper)
   1. Health. 2. Nutrition. 3. Exercise. 4. Diet. I. Title
RA776 .T726 2001
613—dc21   00-054918

To my wonderful William.
You are the essence of my world.

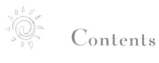

Contents

Introduction

Do you want to increase your odds of living a long, healthy life while staying fit, looking terrific, being socially active, and being mentally and spiritually fulfilled along the way? Of course. Who doesn't? The key to successful longevity, as I call it, is living well every day. It's not just about the length of time you're given on this earth, but the quality of life you live while you're here.

You must realize and accept that your life as you experience it today is a result of the seeds you've planted in your personal garden. The evidence of these long-life seeds of good physical, emotional, and spiritual health, when sown in your youth, will be readily apparent as you enter your forties — or even earlier. I have seen the results of many poorly sown seeds firsthand. I know people in their late thirties who partied hearty and neglected their health and appearance; now they are feeling and looking old long before their time. I also know people in their fifties and sixties who have taken good care of themselves, and as a result look and feel many years younger.

Believe me, Mother Nature will have the last laugh if you don't take steps to preserve what you've got. If you're not happy with what you see in the mirror and how you feel, you can, with knowledge and determination, greatly improve these conditions. It's never too late to initiate a change for the better.

Today, there is so much confusing information about how to eat right, lose weight, be more energetic, look younger, de-stress, and be healthier, that it can leave your head spinning. I'm here to tell you that it's really not all that complicated. It's about getting back to basics, back to simplicity, back into your comfort zone, in tune with what you intuitively know to be right for you. Never forget that you are a unique individual who deserves to look fabulous, live life to the fullest, and feel healthy with every breath you take. You can't simply expect to be physically healthy if you ignore the intellectual, spiritual, social, and emotional sides of your life. Successful longevity demands a life in balance, just as a balanced diet is needed to maintain vitality. Aging is inevitable, but you *can* age beautifully, gracefully, joyfully, and more slowly.

Living a long, vital, robust life, and looking great while doing it, is directly related to sound nutrition, proper exercise and skin care, stress management, a sensible wellness program, a feeling of belonging, and spiritual practice. *How to Feel Fabulous Today!* is written from the heart, so that all women may feel and look truly fabulous all the days of their lives. In this book I share my secrets — sound bits of advice that allow me to work a full schedule with energy to spare, stay fit, maintain my youthful appearance, satisfy my soul, and nourish my spirit. I hope they will add years to your life, life to your years, grace to your body, wisdom to your mind, and peace to your spirit.

Blessings to you and yours.

The strongest principle of growth lies in human choice.

—GEORGE ELIOT

Acknowledgments

I owe much gratitude to my mother,

Brenda Anchors,

and grandmothers,

Phenie Ashe and Grace Anchors,

for their lifelong lessons in beauty,

strength, determination, self-esteem,

spirituality, natural health care,

planting crops by the phases of the moon,

and harvesting and preparing nutritious

and delicious foods.

Their generations of imparted

wisdom have helped make this book

and my life what it is.

I love you all dearly.

Today Is Big with Blessings.

—MARY BAKER EDDY

1

Favor
Feel-Good Foods

Many people take better care of their cars and pets than they do of themselves. They'll put the best and most expensive fuel and oil in their vehicles to ensure top performance and feed their animals brand-name or even home-cooked food to keep them healthy. So why do so many women complain of not feeling well, while feeding themselves substandard fuel? There is a connection, after all.

Your dietary intake, unlike genetics, is a health factor over which you have complete control and which determines, in large part, your energy level, overall appearance, emotional status, mental acuity, and general health, present and future.

A nutrient-rich diet satisfies your body, mind, and soul. Eat some feel-good foods today!

Enjoy More Soy

Soybeans are touted as one of today's miracle foods — and justifiably so. This queen of the bean world is abundant in fiber (unless highly processed), protein, complex carbohydrates, and it contains a moderate amount of healthy fat. Soybeans are a good source of B vitamins, lecithin, iron, potassium, and calcium, and, unlike other beans, they have an almost perfect amino acid profile that is similar to animal protein. They even contain lysine, an amino acid not common to many plant foods.

Soybeans are rich in a group of compounds called phytochemicals, including plant estrogen and isoflavones. These very compounds have a wide range of positive effects on health, such as lowering the risk of heart disease, kidney disease, and cancer, as well as helping to prevent osteoporosis, fighting diabetes, and decreasing the symptoms of menopause.

Soy Many Possibilities

There are many varieties of soy foods available on the market today. Purchase a couple of good soy cookbooks and experiment with all the forms of soy. You may find, to your surprise, that you actually enjoy eating soy, the bean the Chinese call "the meat without bones."

~ **Soybeans.** Cooked at home as a dried bean or purchased canned, soybeans are tasty and full of protein and soluble and insoluble fiber. Unprocessed soybeans are great for diabetics, as the soluble fiber helps maintain stable blood sugar. I like to make soybean burgers — a heart-healthy alternative to greasy hamburgers — from the cooked and mashed beans.

~ **Edamame.** Sold frozen or fresh, edamame are green, unprocessed soybeans that are steamed or boiled for 5 to 10 minutes until tender. They taste like a cross between fresh peas and pinto beans and are very high in protein.

~ **Soybean isolates.** Generally sold as a flavorless powder and commonly found in powdered protein drink mixes or protein energy bars, this form can be used to make delicious protein-rich fruit smoothies and shakes. Add to baking mixes to enhance the protein value.

~ **Toasted soybeans.** Frequently called soy nuts, these have a dry, light crunch and are terrific added to salads in place of croutons. They make a perfect portable snack food, too.

~ **Soymilk.** A super product for those who are allergic to cow's milk. It can be used cup for cup to replace cow's milk as a beverage, over cereal, or in recipes. The flavor of this product varies significantly from manufacturer to manufacturer, so you may have to try a few brands in order to find one you enjoy. It should contain about 6 to 10 grams of protein, 7 to 13 grams of carbohydrates, and 1 to 4 grams of fat per 8-ounce serving. Some brands have lots of added sweeteners (carbohydrates) in an attempt to modify the natural taste, so be sure to read the label carefully if you don't want the extra calories and sugars.

~ **Miso.** A fermented, salty soybean paste used to flavor foods or make a tasty broth base.

~ **Tofu.** This white, flavorless blob, made by curdling and pressing hot soymilk, is actually the ultimate chameleon food. It can assume the taste of whatever dish it is

The Dark Side of Soy

How can a food so healthful and delicious have a downside? According to Pioneer Nutritional Formulas, Inc., publishers of the newsletter *Pioneer Pearls,* soybeans contain five types of plant chemicals that, in sufficient quantities, can be toxic to humans: (1) *soy allergens* may affect up to 20 percent of our population; (2) *phytates* can bind to and prevent absorption of essential minerals; (3) *protease inhibitors* may interfere with the function of protein-digesting pancreatic enzymes; (4) *genistein* can inhibit at least three metabolic pathways needed to maintain normal brain function; and (5) *goitrogens* can latch on to iodine, preventing its absorption.

These compounds are generally present in small quantities so, if you are not allergic, enjoy soy in moderation. Don't overconsume the more processed products, such as soy protein isolates and powders, which may provide undesirable concentrations of soy toxins.

added to and it is available in many textures to suit any dish. Tofu is high in protein and low in carbohydrates, and it contains minimal fiber.

～ **Tempeh.** A tender, fermented, flavorful, high-protein and high-fiber cake of pressed soybeans that is occasionally mixed with other whole grains. It can be sliced or cubed and added to soups and stews or fried and used in vegetarian tortillas.

～ **Soy cheese.** Another tasty boon for the dairy and lactose intolerant. Available in several flavors and textures, soy cheese can be used as a dairy cheese replacement in most recipes. Not all brands of the hard-cheese style melt easily, so try a few. Soy cheese is generally high in protein and low in carbohydrates, but it has no fiber and it varies in fat content.

～ **Soy flour.** A nutritionally dense, heavy flour with a slightly beany flavor. High in protein, moderate in carbohydrates and fat, and high in fiber, it can be used in any recipe calling for wheat flour, except when a light, fluffy texture is desired. Soy flour is usually available lightly toasted to heighten the flavor and improve digestibility.

～ **Textured soy protein.** You've probably eaten this without even knowing it. It's frequently used as a food extender in fast-food hamburgers, side-dish mixes, and in freeze-dried camping/hiking foods. It is produced by pressure-cooking and drying oil-extracted soy flour. It is a complete protein, low in fiber and carbohydrates, and it is available in many varieties. Use textured soy protein as a meat replacement in stews, kabobs, chilis, burgers, and meatloaf recipes.

～ **Soy yogurt.** This plain, unsweetened, off-white yogurt is similar to cow's milk yogurt in texture, but it is a bit more tart; the flavor may take a bit of getting used to. You can eat it straight or use it in recipes as you would regular yogurt. It contains moderate amounts of protein, carbohydrates, and fat, and no fiber.

Eat Organic

Do you really know what you're eating when you bite into a fresh peach, have a side dish of green beans along with a piece of roasted chicken, or enjoy a bowl of ripe, plump strawberries and cream for dessert?

Do you know where the food came from or how it was raised and processed? Unless you're eating certified organically produced food or you purchase food from a local farmer whom you know and trust you don't have a clue.

Eating organically is not a new-fangled idea. It's how your grandparents and great-grandparents ate and raised their food before chemical farming "improved" our foods and growing methods.

Today more than ever, our mass-produced food supply is contaminated with myriad chemicals that have the potential to cause harmful side effects — if not immediately, then in the years ahead. Labeling is not required to inform the public of the particular synthetic fertilizers, herbicides, pesticides, insecticides, antibiotics, or hormones, or to inform of whether the food was irradiated or genetically engineered.

Your health and the health of future generations is a heavy price to pay for this chemical and biological experimentation. For long-term soundness of body and mind, I recommend eating as much certified organically produced food as possible.

Quick Starts

Even though we know we should, most of us have little — if any — time to prepare a nourishing breakfast each and every morning. Cold cereal is quick and so is toast or a bagel, but these aren't always the healthiest choices. Not only do they often lack sufficient protein and fiber, but also they are frequently made from refined grains. They can get boring after a while, too.

Skipping breakfast can lead to junk-food snacking come midmorning when your energy, blood-sugar level, and willpower plummet. To avoid this running-on-empty feeling and keep your engine humming all morning long, breakfast should contain ample protein, filling fiber, minimal refined sugar, and sufficient complex carbohydrates.

Quick and healthy breakfast choices include instant oatmeal topped with a handful of slice almonds and raisins; dried fruit-and-nut trail mix; or 1 cup of low-fat yogurt with a slice of banana. Stick-to-Your-Ribs Peanut Butter Muffins (see page 10) and fresh fruit are also excellent. Yes, breakfast *is* the most important meal of the day.

Stick-to-Your-Ribs Peanut Butter Muffins

As a peanut butter fanatic, I'm always on the look-out for ways to incorporate this nutritious food into my meals. These small, portable, nutritional powerhouse muffins don't contain the poor-quality fat and refined sugar present in most commercial muffins. Make enough muffins on Sunday afternoon for quick breakfasts all week long — perfect for the person on the go.

½ cup date sugar (available in health food stores)

⅔ cup smooth or crunchy organic, room-temperature peanut butter

3 large egg whites or equivalent egg substitute

1½ teaspoons vanilla extract

2½ cups organic whole-wheat flour or wheat-free pancake and waffle mix

1 tablespoon oat bran or wheat bran

1 cup yogurt or soy yogurt

½ cup plus 2 tablespoons low-fat or nonfat cow's milk or soymilk

½ cup chopped unsalted roasted peanuts (optional)

1. Preheat oven to 400°F. Coat 12 standard muffin pan cups with nonstick

cooking spray or use paper muffin cup liners.

2. In a large bowl, using an electric mixer or a spoon, beat together date sugar and peanut butter until well blended. Beat in egg whites, then vanilla.

3. In another large bowl, fold the flour or dry mix, bran, yogurt, and milk together until blended. Gradually add this mixture to the peanut butter mixture until moistened. Divide batter evenly among prepared muffin cups. *Optional*: Sprinkle each muffin top with 2 teaspoons of chopped peanuts.

4. Bake until tops are lightly browned and a toothpick inserted into center of muffin comes out clean, about 15–18 minutes. Be careful not to overbake or the muffins will be dry. Remove muffins from pan as soon as possible and transfer to wire rack to cool completely — though they're also delicious hot and slathered with even more peanut butter!

Yield: 12 muffins

Age-Defying Antioxidants

The media is abuzz these days about the dangers of free radicals and the benefits of antioxidants, but do you actually know what these terms mean? *Free radicals* are those pesky molecules with unpaired electrons in their outer shell that accelerate the aging process by damaging cells. The majority naturally occur in the body and are produced as a by-product of normal cellular activity, and some are also generated by physical and psychological stress.

Free radicals are increasingly found in our environment in the form of pollution, radiation, and chemical agents — such as pesticides, herbicides, insecticides, and synthetic fertilizers — in and on our foods. Smoked, fried, or barbecued meats, a high-fat diet, coffee, soda, and alcohol are additional sources. Free radicals are responsible for many of the symptoms and diseases often associated with aging, such as wrinkles, age spots, skin cancer, arthritis, osteoporosis, arteriosclerosis, scleroderma, cataracts, memory loss, weakened immune system, and diabetes, among others.

Antioxidants are the soldiers in the battle against free radicals. How do antioxidants work? Think of what happens when you cut a fresh apple in half and let it sit on the counter — it turns brown, or oxidizes. But if you squirt the apple with lemon juice, an antioxidant, immediately after cutting the fruit turns brown much more slowly. That's what antioxidants do to your body — they slow down the aging, or oxidation, process. Definitely a good thing.

Your first line of defense is to consume a diet rich in antioxidant compounds, such as vitamins C and E, beta-carotene, and the phytochemicals (quercetin, flavonoids, lycopene, and ellagic acid). Try to include at least 3 to 5 servings of vegetables and 2 to 4 servings of fruits a day to receive the most benefit. Some ideas for antioxidant-rich foods appear below.

Supplements should be used only to augment your diet, not to replace a variety of plant-based foods. Foods, unlike supplements, supply vital combinations of nutrients that work synergistically with each other, nourishing the body in ways not yet completely understood.

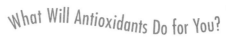

What Will Antioxidants Do for You?

Elizabeth Somer, author of *Age-Proof Your Body: Your Complete Guide to Lifelong Vitality* explains it this way:

> While you can't peek into your cells to judge the war's outcome, you can get a frontline report by how you feel and look. A well-stocked antioxidant system will help maintain a youthful appearance, healthy body, and clear mind. Numerous studies report that people who consume ample amounts of antioxidants from either food or supplements and maintain high blood levels of these nutrients also are the least likely to develop heart disease, cancer, cataracts, arthritis, and other diseases.

Eating for Youthful Vitality

In addition to being chock-full of antioxidants, the foods listed below are nutritional all-stars. They're low in fat, sodium, and calories (with the exception of nuts and seeds); contain no cholesterol; are excellent sources of fiber; and supply age-defying minerals, such as magnesium, boron, selenium, iron, calcium, and potassium. Incorporate these foods in your diet every day.

⁓ **Berries:** grapes and grape juice, blackberries, blueberries, bilberries, cranberries, strawberries, boysenberries, and mulberries

⁓ **Tea:** black and green teas

⁓ **Melons:** cantaloupe, watermelon, honeydew, and Crenshaw

⁓ **Vegetables:** red or green loose-leaf, Boston, and romaine lettuce, mesclun mixes, spinach, broccoli, Brussels sprouts, kale, carrots, tomatoes, bell peppers (red, orange, and yellow), string beans, cabbage, onions, garlic, potatoes, and celery

⁓ **Tree fruits:** apples, apricots, peaches, cherries, bananas, pears, kiwis, citrus, and plums

⁓ **Nuts and seeds:** almonds, Brazil nuts, walnuts, pecans, sesame and sunflower seeds

⁓ **Legumes:** pinto, black turtle, soy, lima, great northern, kidney, navy, and all types of peas

Simple Ways to Add More Fruits and Veggies to Your Diet

Did you know that most people in the United States do not consume the basic daily dietary recommendations of fruits and vegetables? According to the National Health Association, only 10 percent of the population eats the daily USDA Food Guide Pyramid's *minimum* recommendation of 5 servings of fruits and vegetables each day. Eleven percent consume no fruits or vegetables in any given day, 45 percent of adults consume no fruits per day, and 22 percent of adults consume no vegetables per day. Surprised? So was I!

Eating less than the recommended amounts of these food groups can leave you deficient in fiber, vitamins, minerals, important immunity-boosting antioxidants, and cancer-protecting phytochemicals. Fruits and vegetables fill you up, not out, which is a boon to your waistline, too. Today many nutritionists advise that you even increase the Pyramid's serving recommendations to 3 to 5 fruits per day and at least 4 to 8 vegetables per day. Don't be a statistic — eat more fruits and vegetables!

Not sure how to integrate all those servings into your daily diet? Follow my recommendations below for 12 easy ways to eat more health-promoting produce.

12 Easy Ways to Eat More Produce

1. Freeze small chunks of bananas, strawberries, pears, melons, mangos, or peaches in resealable freezer bags and add to fruit smoothies for a refreshing snack or quick breakfast.
2. Make vegetable kabobs and cook on the grill.
3. Take a large bag of raw veggies to work every day for low-calorie finger food. It sure beats hitting the vending machine or doughnut shop for a snack.
4. Make frozen fruit kabobs and serve as a light snack or refreshing dessert.
5. Drink vegetable juice (available at health food stores or make your own) instead of soda or fruit juice drinks.
6. Keep a colorful fruit salad in your refrigerator at all times for convenient, healthy nibbling.
7. Keep bags of dried fruits in your purse and car.

8. Be adventurous! Try one new fruit or vegetable each week.

9. Experiment with international vegetarian recipes that include lots of flavorful vegetable combinations and use interesting herbs and spices.

10. Eat whole fruit for breakfast or double the amount you ordinarily add to your bowl of cereal or porridge.

11. Enjoy delicious cold fruit soup or gazpacho as a light lunch or appetizer.

12. Cook a big pot of vegetarian chili or stew accompanied by a chunk of hearty, whole-grain bread.

EFAs: Essentials for Well-Being

Lowfat, nonfat, bad fat, trans-fat: sounds like a Dr. Seuss book. Since the early 1980s, the dietary dictum has been to avoid just about all fatty foods because they are high in calories. Indeed they are, but what we failed to understand was that a little healthy fat is necessary for proper functioning of many bodily processes. Now multitudes of people are paying the price for this fat phobia. A deficiency of essential fatty acids (EFAs) can lead to arthritis, joint stiffness, acne, dry skin, eczema, slow healing, diarrhea, and hair loss, among other things. Most nutrition experts recommend that 15 to 25 percent of your daily caloric intake should consist of fats, provided that the bulk of those calories come in the form of beneficial unsaturated fats.

An extremely low-fat diet, a diet high in saturated fat, and a diet that includes lots of refined foods containing trans-fatty acids are all detrimental to your health. Trans-fatty acids, which are identified on labels with the words *hydrogenated oil* or *partially hydrogenated oil* should be avoided like the plague. This type of fat is found in many of the processed convenience foods we eat, such as cookies, cakes, chips, doughnuts, breads, shortening, ready-made pie crust, muffin/cookie mixes, pizza, and some prepackaged side dishes (like rice, noodles, and potatoes).

"Feel-Good" Fats and Their Benefits

Esssential fatty acids have been conspicuously absent from our diets. As the name suggests, these fats are essential for optimal bodily functioning, but because they are not produced by the body they must be supplied in the diet or via supplements. Here are some suggestions for foods containing the important omega-3 and omega-6 fatty acids. Follow label directions or the advice of your health care professional when adding any of these supplements and foods to your diet.

~ **Flaxseeds.** Two tablespoons daily of pure, buttery-tasting, expeller-pressed, unfiltered flaxseed oil poured over your salad, used as a dip for bread, or taken straight, has been shown to help fight dry skin, itchy scalp, dandruff, arthritic symptoms, dry hair, arthritis, allergies, immune deficiencies, constipation, and poor eyesight and color perception. Flaxseeds are high in omega-3 fatty acids and lignans, phytonutrients that support immune function. Ground flaxseeds are good sprinkled over salads, too.

~ **Healthful oils.** Evening primrose oil, borage oil, and the less potent black currant oil can be taken daily in capsule form. I take one or two 1,300 mg capsules of evening primrose oil each day to ease the symptoms of premenstrual syndrome (PMS), keep dry skin at bay, and make my hair shiny. These oils are rich in omega-6 fatty acids, which are necessary for fluid balance, blood clotting, hormone synthesis, nerve function, strong immune function, and prevention of cardiovascular disease.

Cod liver oil, high in omega-3 fatty acids, taken in capsule form or as a flavored oil (I like the orange flavor), is great for stiff joints, dry skin, and arthritis. My mother-in-law swears by this stuff; she calls it her "youthifying" oil, noting that it keeps her skin smooth and moisturized and it's the reason she rarely gets sick.

~ **Blue-green algae.** Blue-green algae contains high levels of omega-6 fatty acids and beta-carotene and can be of great benefit for people suffering from skin disorders, such as acne, psoriasis, and eczema. I add a couple of teaspoons of blue-green algae powder to my daily green drink. It has been a real help in healing any bouts of stress-induced adult acne and severe PMS symptoms.

~ **Nuts.** For a healthful, nutrient-dense snack with omega-3 fatty acids, grab a handful of raw walnuts or Brazil nuts or chop them and add to your salads. They add crunchiness in lieu of croutons.

~ **Cold-water fish.** Two to three servings per week of cold-water fish are recommended to obtain sufficient omega-3 fatty acids. In my opinion, bluefish and mackerel are best eaten within hours of being caught; otherwise they can taste a bit on the strong,

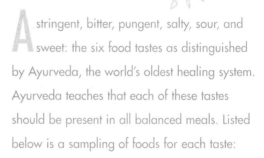

The Six Tastes of Food

Astringent, bitter, pungent, salty, sour, and sweet: the six food tastes as distinguished by Ayurveda, the world's oldest healing system. Ayurveda teaches that each of these tastes should be present in all balanced meals. Listed below is a sampling of foods for each taste:

~ **Astringent:** Apples, beans, black tea, blackberries, cabbage, lentils, oak bark tea, persimmons, potatoes, yellow dock (herbal) tea.

~ **Bitter:** Greens such as chicory, dandelion, endive, radicchio, sorrel; gentian (herbal) tea; kale, rhubarb, spinach.

fishy side. Cod, a white-fleshed fish, is available in most seafood markets; it is mild tasting and is enjoyed by people who prefer a blander variety of fish. Salmon and tuna, on the pricey side if purchased fresh, are available canned and can be made into patties, salads, and sandwiches, and served hot or cold.

⁓ **Pungent:** Cayenne, jalapeño, and habanero peppers; elecampane or peppermint (herbal) tea; garlic, ginger, onions, radishes.

⁓ **Salty:** Seaweed, salt.

⁓ **Sour:** Fermented foods, such as aged cheese, Chinese sour plums, pickles, yogurt, lemons, vinegar.

⁓ **Sweet:** Chocolate, corn, most dairy products, honey, meats, medjool dates, oils, rice, sugar, wheat, yams.

Challenge yourself to create menus that are balanced in nutrition and taste, then enjoy them regularly.

Wonderful Water

Water is a powerful, life-giving element. The body is approximately 70 to 80 percent water, and although you can live without food for maybe 6 weeks, without water you could survive for only about 8 to 10 days.

Water is necessary for cellular function, helping to control body temperature, lubricate joints, and aid digestion and nutrient transportation. It is also the main component of our blood. But according to Dr. Fereydoon Batmanghelidj, M.D., author of *Your Body's Many Cries for Water*, chronic dehydration is the root of many of the health problems the world is experiencing today. These include heartburn, rheumatoid joint pain, back pain, angina, migraine headaches, colitis, asthma, high blood pressure, and constipation. Dr. Batmanghelidj states that the body indicates its water shortage by producing pain.

Keep in mind that thirst is not always the best indicator that it's time for a drink. The sensation of thirst usually means that you're dehydrated and long overdue for several glasses of water.

Liquid Assets

Water can be a powerful factor in maximizing your health, so make sure you're drinking enough water each day by following these important hydration tips:

~ **Drink at least 8 cups of water per day, more if you're active.** Coffee, caffeinated tea, alcoholic drinks (including wine and beer), and sodas don't count toward your total. In fact, you should drink an additional cup of water for each cup of caffeinated or alcoholic beverage consumed.

~ **Increase water consumption if ill or dieting and before and after any vigorous activity.** This includes any activity that requires intense mental concentration. To rehydrate yourself in a hurry, the best drink is water at room temperature.

~ **Make water consumption routine.** Keep a water pitcher on your office desk, a bottle in your car, a bottle in your gym bag, and a small container in your purse. A half hour before each meal, consume 1 to 2 cups to curb your appetite and enhance digestion.

~ **Liquid fuel.** Did you know that you can work out for significantly less time than those people who drink water before, during, and after exercise? Slight dehydration can even cause aerobic capacity to decrease.

— **Hidden thirst?** You may think you're hungry when you're really just thirsty. Next time you've got the munchies, drink a cup of ice-cold water, wait a few minutes, and see if your food craving doesn't disappear. Regularly drinking water will keep your stomach full and hunger to a minimum.

— **Eliminate the bloat.** When you don't drink your daily quota of water, your body intelligently secretes aldosterone, a hormone that prompts tissues to retain water, thus causing that puffy, waterlogged appearance and sluggish feeling.

Eat Your Medicine

Did you know that many medicinal herbs are both tasty and nutritious? Forget the notion that herbal medicine consists only of bad-tasting brews, foul-flavored tinctures, bitter pills and capsules, and gritty powders. Fresh, full-of-flavor herbs are easy to grow in pots or in your garden plot and can also be found in wild meadows or woodlands.

I'm not talking about the standard culinary herbs, such as tarragon, oregano, basil, marjoram, or rosemary; I'm talking about often ignored "wild foods" or "herbal weeds" that can make a substantial yet inexpensive addition to your daily intake of easily assimilable nutrients.

Take a Walk on the Wild Side

Depending on your local climate, fresh, wild food and beverage herbs can be grown from seed or wild-harvested almost year-round except during the coldest winter months. (See Resources for seed sources.) I have listed only those wild foods that are commonly found throughout the country and offer you the widest spectrum of flavor, vitamins, minerals, and phytochemicals.

~ **Dandelion** *(Taraxacum officinale).* This lowly bitter "weed" should be part of everyone's diet. The root and leaf are rich sources of vitamins A, B, and C, as well as calcium, potassium, iron, and other trace minerals. It is a great spring tonic herb that revitalizes stagnant winter blood and enhances liver function and digestion. It's terrific as a salad herb, and the young flowers are edible, too. Mild-flavored dandelion tea (made from dried root and leaves) acts as a gentle laxative and mineral supplement.

~ **Lamb's-quarters** *(Chenopodium album)*. A mild-flavored herb that is sometimes called "wild spinach," lamb's-quarters may be eaten raw in salads or steamed like spinach. It doesn't usually become bitter with maturity, therefore it may be harvested throughout the growing season. This herb is high in protein, iron, phosphorus, calcium, and vitamins A and C.

~ **Stinging nettle** *(Urtica dioica)*. A prickly, irritating herb best purchased in dried form and consumed as a tasty beverage tea. The young, tender shoots and new top growth can also be harvested if you wear gloves. Then steam the herb until tender to destroy the irritating formic acid. Nettle is amazingly high in vitamin A, calcium, and easily assimilable iron.

~ **Purslane** *(Portulaca oleracea)*. Prostrate growing and fleshy leafed, purslane often invades my garden and annual flower beds. A favorite addition to my summer salads, this mild-flavored "weed" has high levels of vitamins A and C and lesser amounts of calcium and phosphorus. Eat it raw or steamed.

～ **Chickweed** *(Stellaria media)*. This common lawn "weed" has diminutive, white, starlike flowers that add interest as a salad ingredient. It is mildly flavored and chock-full of vitamins A and C with lesser amounts of silicon, sulfur, manganese, copper, zinc, phosphorus, chromium, and selenium. Chickweed also acts as a mineral-rich diuretic, especially if 2 to 3 cups of mild tea are taken daily as needed. I find that it helps relieve excess bloat during PMS or after excess sodium intake.

～ **Nasturtium** *(Tropaeolum majus)*. A native South American plant that contains vitamins A and C, iron, trace minerals, and a small amount of sodium. Nasturtium's flower buds can be eaten pickled as "poor man's capers" in your salad. Consumption of the entire plant is beneficial for breaking up congestion.

～ **Watercress** *(Nasturtium officinale)*. A hot and spicy little green herb that contains plenty of calcium, potassium, magnesium, manganese, copper, zinc, iodine, phosphorus, and vitamins A and E. Watercress makes an interesting addition to cucumber and tomato sandwiches and salads.

~ **Violet (*Viola odorata* and related spp.).** Mild tasting leaves with beautiful edible flowers that are white, lavender, or dark

Rules for Harvesting Wild Herbs

If growing your "wild food" in pots or in your organic garden, obviously adhere only to those rules that pertain to your circumstances.

~ **Harvest ethically.** Pick only those plants that are growing in abundance. If you overharvest an area, plants can't regenerate the next year.

~ **Pick fresh.** Harvest only plants that are young, fresh, and tender. Wild foods, especially greens, tend to get tough and bitter as they mature.

~ **Know what you're doing.** Always check with the property owner before entering a property and picking their "wild weeds," and

purple. Like nasturtiums, violet flowers make elegant additions to your salads, and they leave your mouth tasting like flowers, too. The young leaf is very high in vitamins A and C and can be eaten raw or steamed.

by all means heed No TRESPASSING signs. Have a wild plant field guide in hand while harvesting to avoid picking a similar-looking plant that may be poisonous.

⁓ **Avoid contaminated plants.** Petrochemicals, exhaust fumes, lawn chemicals, weed killers, and animal excrement are problematic along busy roadsides, congested neighborhoods, and some farmlands. Avoid harvesting plants from these areas.

⁓ **Clean well.** Thoroughly wash, and scrub when appropriate, all edible plant parts prior to eating. Make sure to look for bugs and extra debris not commonly found in grocery store produce.

It's Easy Being Green

According to Susan Smith Jones, Ph.D., author of *Choose Radiant Health & Happiness*, "All life on this planet is derived either directly or indirectly from the sunlight that falls on chlorophyll. Chlorophyll is the green pigment found in plants, algae, and fresh dark green vegetables. . . . Some of the best sources of nutrients that prevent disease and support health are found in plants that are rich in green color, and one of the reasons is the color itself."

Chlorophyll's chemical structure is similar to hemoglobin, the iron-containing pigment in our blood. Chlorophyll has the ability to raise the red blood-cell count, thus infusing our blood with more oxygen and increasing circulation — which results in more energy, efficient removal of waste, and more rapid cell proliferation that speeds healing processes. This green pigment also reduces body and breath odor.

Green foods, or *super foods* as they're sometimes called, refer to a group of water and land-based plants that contain high levels of chlorophyll, complex carbohydrates, amino acids, vitamins (in particular beta-carotene and B-complex), minerals (including important trace minerals), enzymes, and other vital nutrients.

Remember that green foods supplements are just that: supplements. They are not a replacement for a diet rich in vegetables, fruits, and whole grains.

The following green dietary supplements are freshly harvested, freeze dried, and then either encapsulated, formed into tablets, or sold as supplemental powders. Many health food stores with juice bars will offer freshly extracted wheatgrass juice, which tastes like freshly mown grass to me.

Grassy Greens

~ **Barley grass.** This is my favorite of the grasses because of its sweet flavor. I add one heaping tablespoon of powder to a glass of tomato juice each morning and drink it on an empty stomach. It takes the edge off my appetite and energizes me.

~ **Wheatgrass.** The original green food supplement, wheatgrass is very similar to barley grass in nutritional content. It's easy to grow organically at home in trays for juicing.

~ **Alfalfa.** Grown primarily as feed for the livestock industry, alfalfa is actually a leguminous plant with a very, very long taproot that reaches deep into mineral-rich soil. It is similar to the other grasses in nutritional content, but it has the flavor of newly mown hay.

Fresh-Water Microalgae

~ **Chlorella.** A more complex algae that is exceptionally rich in chlorophyll; it provides the highest percent of almost any plant. It's also very high in vitamin B_{12}. Tastes a bit "fishy," like all algae.

~ **Blue-green algae.** Structurally, these are the simplest of the algae. Blue-green algae contain high levels of beta-carotene, B-complex vitamins, and protein. Spirulina is one species of blue-green algae, and it is often cultivated in man-made ponds utilizing fresh and/or salt water and added nutrients to facilitate growth.

~ **Aphanizomenon flos-aqua (AFA).** Another species of blue-green algae, this type may contain higher levels of naturally-occurring nutrients, especially gamma linolenic acid (GLA) and vitamin K.

2
Work toward Wellness

Wellness is no longer limited to a trip to the psychiatrist or physician. Today, wellness is the desired end of a multifaceted journey that benefits from myriad ancient, traditional, and modern health-care therapies. Being well means being whole, connected — a smooth-running sum of individual parts. A disturbance in one part of your being means that the other components are not working up to par, either.

Although in this chapter I focus on a few specific problems that are especially important to your basic physical health, I also offer glimpses into aromatherapy, reiki, stress reduction, and massage. These avenues offer emotional and spiritual support that, when incorporated into a total wellness package, will bring your body, mind, and spirit into balance and wellness.

Aromatherapy for Body, Mind, and Home

Lately the word *aromatherapy* leaves a bad taste in my mouth. In the name of commercialism and profits, it's become tainted. Seems everyone in the industry who utilizes fragrances in their products slaps *aromatherapy* on their label to increase sales and tells you that the aromatic ingredient(s) contained within will whisk away your cares and physical problems with a mere whiff. Hogwash! The term is being applied to a vast array of products ranging from cheap grocery-store scented candles, bubble bath, air fresheners, and carpet cleaners to expensive salon shampoos and cosmetics. I

Know This

Vegetable oils, synthetic fragrance oils, and inferior diluted essential oils have an oily texture and leave an oily residue. Pure essential oils are highly volatile, evaporate relatively quickly, and have no oily residue or texture.

can guarantee you that most of these products contain synthetic fragrance oils and/or inferior quality, highly refined essential oils whose fragrance will temporarily tantalize your nose, but contribute nothing toward healing your psyche, easing your physical illness, or cleaning your home environment.

True, effective aromatherapy utilizes real, minimally refined pure essential oils that are of pharmaceutical and aromatherapeutic grade, and they are often processed from plants that are organically raised or ethically wildcrafted. The practice of aromatherapy has scientific roots. The various chemical components in each particular essential oil have been studied to see how their usage can affect the body on an emotional and physiological level. Many essential oils also contain antiseptic and degreasing qualities, which make them superb household cleansing additives. To guide and educate you in this fascinating mind/body healing modality, I suggest that you purchase an aromatherapy book that outlines the properties and uses of essential oils. See the Recommended Readings for book suggestions, and see the Resources for reputable essential oil companies.

Essential Oil Precautions

Essential oils are highly concentrated natural products and must be used with caution. To test for potential allergic reactions, try this patch test.

1. In a small bowl, combine 1 or 2 drops of the essential oil in question and 1 teaspoon base oil (vegetable oil or nut oil).

2. Apply a dab of the mixture to the underside of your wrist, the inside of your upper arm, behind your ear, or behind your knee. Wait 24 hours.

3. If no irritation develops after 24 hours, the oil in question is generally safe for you to use. If irritation develops, do *not* use the oil.

11 Basic Essential Oils

The following essential oils have many uses and should be included in the family medicine and cosmetic cabinets. I highly recommend that you use a few of these oils to replace harsh, environmentally unsound household cleansing products.

~ **Clove** *(Syzygium aromaticum)*. A strong antibacterial, analgesic, and antiseptic. It is best known as a cure for toothaches. Place a single drop on the offending tooth and surrounding gum area for fast, temporary relief of pain — then see your dentist. Clove can also be used, like orange and lemon essential oils, in household cleansing formulas.

~ **Eucalyptus** *(Eucalyptus globulus)*. This deeply penetrating, camphorous oil is a must-have if you're suffering from a head cold or respiratory infection. For relief of stuffiness and congested lungs, boil 4 cups of water, then remove from heat. Add 6 drops essential oil, make a tent over your head and pot with a towel, and inhale the healing vapors for 10 minutes. Be sure to close your eyes and avoid touching the hot pot.

~ **Lavender** *(Lavandula angustifolia)*. A mild multipurpose oil that smells like an old-fashioned floral perfume. Simply inhaling this oil calms the mind, relaxes the body, and soothes the spirit. This antiseptic healing oil should be kept in every kitchen as a burn remedy. Immediately after receiving a burn, immerse the affected area in cold water or cold aloe vera gel, then apply a thin layer of lavender essential oil. It will assist in rapid skin cell regeneration and help keep scarring to a minimum.

~ **Lemon** *(Citrus limon)*. Has a familiar clean, fresh, invigorating scent. Use in the same applications as orange essential oil, mentioned above. This oil is also beneficial for oily, acneic skin because of its astringent, antibacterial, and antiseptic properties. Add 10 drops to 1 cup of witch hazel extract, shake well, and use as a toner to remove excess sebum and residue after cleansing your skin.

~ **Moroccan blue chamomile** *(Tanacetum annuum)*. This is a blessing for those suffering from itchy, rashy, dry, or inflamed skin, as well as hives and poison oak or ivy. I like to add 10 drops to a 2-ounce container of skin cream and apply to affected areas as necessary. You may also use this blend as a daily facial moisturizer to keep the skin clear and supple.

~ **Orange** *(Citrus sinensis)*. This oil is a great degreaser. You can also add 10 drops of essential oil to 8 ounces of witch hazel for an oily skin toner. Shake well before each use.

 ∽ **Peppermint** *(Mentha piperita).* One of my favorites! Place a drop on your tongue as a breath freshener, or add a drop to a cup of peppermint tea for prompt indigestion relief. For an invigorating, stimulating antidandruff shampoo, add 20 drops to 8 ounces of quality natural shampoo; shake well, then shampoo as usual. It will leave your scalp feeling cool and tingly. To awaken a dull brain in midafternoon, inhale deeply directly from the bottle a few times.

 ∽ **Rose geranium** *(Pelargonium graveolens).* Smells like a rose garden. I like to inhale the aroma directly from the bottle when I feel the need for revitalization. The oil has a balancing quality and helps relieve mental stress and fatigue.

 ∽ **Rosemary** *(Rosmarinus officinalis).* The verbenon chemotype is a terrific oil to stimulate your mind as well as your circulation. Add 20 drops to 8 ounces of moisturizing shower/bath gel or body lotion, shake well, and apply as usual. This antiseptic oil acts as a skin-cell regenerative and wound healer and opens sinus passages.

~ **Tea tree** *(Melaleuca alternifolia)*. A powerful yet gentle-on-the-skin antiviral, antifungal, and broad-spectrum antibacterial. To prevent or heal infection, apply a drop directly to scrapes, scratches, acne pimples, boils, or insect bites. For toenail fungus, apply a drop to affected toe(s) daily until healed. (Fungus is stubborn and difficult to eradicate. This treatment may take several months to remedy the problem. Consistent application is key.)

~ **Thyme** *(Thymus vulgaris)*. The linalol chemotype is a powerful — yet gentle to the skin — antiviral, antibiotic, and antiseptic, I recommend keeping the oil around during cold and flu season. Add a few drops to your vaporizer to cleanse and purify the air or purchase a nebulizing diffuser to slowly release the volatile oils into the surrounding atmosphere. Put a few drops onto a damp sponge before wiping down bathroom and kitchen surfaces; it will kill germs.

To help dry and heal pimples, combine 1 drop of thyme essential oil with ¼ teaspoon of aloe vera juice. Then dab on each pimple with a cotton swab.

All-Purpose Citrus Cleanser

Use this general, all-purpose cleanser for greasy hands and dirty bath and shower stalls, ceramic tiles, sinks, or ovens.

> 1 cup soap flakes
> 1 cup borax
> 1 cup baking soda
> 2 teaspoons orange essential oil

1. In a medium-sized bowl, mix the flakes, borax, and baking soda.
2. Slowly add the essential oil, one drop at a time, stirring to incorporate. Store in a tightly sealed container.
3. To use, blend a tablespoon or more of the formula in a small bowl with enough water to form a slushy texture. Use it to wash hands or scrub bathroom or kitchen surfaces. Rinse with water.

Yield: 3 cups

Aromatherapeutic Massage: Scentual Healing

It's no secret that human touch is powerful. From infants to the elderly and all ages and sizes in between, everyone needs touch in order to thrive. It is reassuring, comforting, energizing, and, many believe — quite rightly — healing.

For many, the word *massage* brings to mind pampering, a luxury few can afford on a daily, weekly, or even monthly basis. In this day and age, a bit of daily pampering is just the ticket to unwind from the day's hectic pace. If you have a willing partner, a daily back, shoulder, neck, scalp, or foot massage is guaranteed to put your relationship on a new level and you in a less stressed mood. Self-massage is another option, but I feel that trading massages with a partner is more beneficial. As a treat, try to get a full-body professional massage at least twice a year. Massage gift certificates make a great gift for a dear friend or spouse.

The power of massage is universally recognized and is one of the most widely practiced complementary therapies, with Swedish massage being the most common form. It relaxes muscles (thereby easing aches and pains), stretches the ligaments and tendons, and improves circulation (helping to shorten recovery time from muscular strain by flushing the tissues of metabolic wastes). The skin and nervous system also benefit from increased blood flow.

During a massage, the therapist applies pressure to the layers of muscles, generally rubbing in the direction of the heart to promote blood flow. The traditional manipulative techniques can be slow and gentle or firm and vigorous depending on the desired results.

There are many different types of massage. *Shiatsu*, a Japanese acupressure massage, involves work on pressure points. *Trigger point massage* is a pain-relief technique geared towards particular tender areas where muscles have been damaged or to relieve spasms and cramping. *Sports massage* is designed to reduce injuries, provide warm-up for athletes before exercise, and help alleviate inflammation. *Rolfing* involves vigorous deep tissue massage that attempts to align the body segments through connective tissue manipulation, and the *Feldenkrais method* uses gentle, hands-on manipulation to improve body alignment and breathing; the practitioner also gives instruction on mental imagery and proper movement.

Beneficial Essential Oils

~ **Stimulating:** basil, black pepper, eucalyptus, lemon, lemongrass, peppermint, pine, sage, rosemary, thyme

~ **Refreshing:** basil, bergamot, cypress, fir, geranium, juniper, lemon, lemongrass, lime, mandarin orange, peppermint, petitgrain, pine, rosemary

~ **Warming:** benzoin, black pepper, cajeput, chamomile, cinnamon, clary sage, clove, coriander, ginger, marjoram, myrrh

~ **Relaxing:** benzoin, cedarwood, chamomile, clary sage, frankincense, geranium, jasmine, lavender, neroli, patchouli, rose, ylang ylang

~ **Headache and sinus congestion:** basil, eucalyptus globulus, lavender, peppermint

~ **Respiration:** cedarwood, eucalyptus globulus, peppermint, pine, ravensara

~ **Stiffness:** cardamom, eucalyptus citriodora, ginger, helichrysum, lavender, marjoram, rosemary

~ **Reproductive balance:** balsam fir, clary sage, geranium, lemon, rose maroc

Aromatherapy massage is the combination of touch and smell, and provides the ultimate feel-fabulous therapy. The power of smell can dramatically affect the mind and emotions via the olfactory nerves in the brain, which are in direct contact with the limbic system. This integration of aromatherapy and touch is effective for creating a mood or to help heal a specific condition.

Custom-Blended Massage Oil

Massage oils can be customized to relax, invigorate, or heal with the addition of pure essential oils. They can be blended to benefit your skin type, as well.

Note: *If you are pregnant, avoid basil, bergamot, cinnamon, clary sage, clove, coriander, eucalyptus, juniper, lemon, lime, marjoram, myrrh, mandarin orange, black pepper, peppermint, pine, ravensara, rosemary, sage, and thyme.*

¼ cup unscented soybean, almond, apricot, hazelnut, or grapeseed oil for base

Up to 15 drops (if skin is sensitive, limit to 6 to 8 drops) of any of the essential oils listed on page 46, singly or in combination

In a 2-ounce dark glass bottle, combine base oil with essential oil(s). Cap tightly. Shake thoroughly before each use. Use as much or as little to achieve desired "slip" or friction on the skin's surface when performing a massage. May be used daily.

Yield: Approximately 2 ounces

Osteoporosis: The Silent Disease

Osteoporosis is a condition of weak, thin, porous bones, and it is not limited to frail, little old ladies anymore. Porous bones can be found in just about anyone, from a 16-year-old football player to a 60-year-old man who's been on prednisone to treat asthma complications.

Osteoporosis is often called the "silent disease" because bone fractures and breaks can occur without warning. Often it's the arm, wrist, or hip that breaks. The bones of the spine are also a common area of thinning. Frequently, over several years or even decades, the supportive vertebrae will collapse upon themselves, causing the trademark stooping posture, loss of height, and back and neck pain.

Bone is a dynamic, living tissue. Like your skin, it is in a continual state of flux, always regenerating and degenerating. This constant tearing down and rebuilding of bone helps keep your skeleton strong.

Bone health is dependent on more than just calcium intake. Maintaining bone

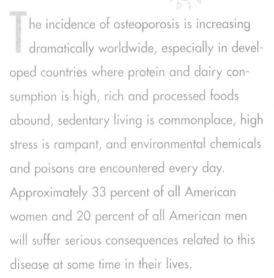

Osteoporosis on the Rise

The incidence of osteoporosis is increasing dramatically worldwide, especially in developed countries where protein and dairy consumption is high, rich and processed foods abound, sedentary living is commonplace, high stress is rampant, and environmental chemicals and poisons are encountered every day. Approximately 33 percent of all American women and 20 percent of all American men will suffer serious consequences related to this disease at some time in their lives.

health is not as simple as popping a daily calcium supplement or drinking a cup of milk. Bone health is determined by the interrelationship of circulating levels of minerals, trace minerals, hormones, vitamins, proteins, and other nutrients, as well as regular weight-bearing activities and sunlight.

Build Better Bones

"The causes of calcium loss may include decreased estrogen in women after menopause, decreased testosterone in elderly men, lack of weight-bearing activity, smoking, dietary animal protein, salt, caffeine, and soda pop. In other words, most instances of osteoporosis are due to lifestyle choices," according to Ronald G. Cridland, M.D., certified member of the International Association of Hygienic Physicians (IAHP). Other causes of osteoporosis can include regular use of steroids and aluminum-containing antacids, lack of regular menses, history of anorexia, low bone density, poor dietary habits, hyperthyroidism, and poor health in general.

Osteoporosis does not have to be a fact of life. It can be prevented to a great degree and is often partially reversible with proper diet, exercise, and lifestyle changes. Disease prevention is always the preferred way to go, but it's never too late to take corrective action no matter the status of your present bone health. Here are some tips to help all adults slow and/or prevent bone loss:

~ **Strengthen your digestion.** Many Americans suffer from poor digestion. Maximum nutrient absorption is not possible with an impaired digestive system, which tends to get worse as you age. See Digest with Ease (page 70) for a more in-depth discussion of your digestive system and ways to improve its functioning.

~ **Moderate your protein intake.** According to John A. McDougall, M.D., "Excess consumption of protein triggers the kidneys to excrete calcium from the body. For people on high-protein diets, these losses are significant. Studies have shown that the quantities of protein commonly consumed by Americans cause calcium to be lost from the body at a rate that is greater than the body's capacity to absorb more calcium. It is estimated that between 1 percent and 4 percent of the adult skeleton is lost each year on the high-animal-protein American diet. This net loss of calcium occurs even when people consume high quantities of calcium."

~ **Eat a "strong bone" diet.** Include plenty of whole grains, fruits, vegetables, nuts, seeds, and canned salmon and sardines and their edible bones, as well as small amounts of organic chicken, pork, beef, and fish. Eliminate processed foods. A strong, supportive skeleton needs plenty of vitamins C, D, K, and calcium, magnesium, manganese, copper, zinc, silicon, boron, moderate amounts of phosphorous, and fluoride.

~ **Moderate dairy intake.** Contrary to popular belief, dairy products are not the best foods for building bones. Yes, most dairy products are high in calcium, but they are also high in protein and leave an acidic ash in the body after digestion. This causes calcium to be excreted from the body, not retained. Additionally, after age 4, most people cannot properly digest dairy products due to an absence of necessary enzyme production. Cow's milk is best suited for calves, not humans.

~ **Make an impact.** Your bones need at least 30 minutes of daily weight-bearing exercise in order to build and preserve the most bone. Brisk walking, stair climbing, weight lifting, running, dancing, and jumping rope fill the bill. A sedentary lifestyle will rapidly accelerate bone loss.

~ **Don't smoke.** Cigarette smoking can inhibit bone growth, boost calcium excretion, and impair digestion. It also slows the healing of fractured or broken bones.

~ **Limit salt and sodas.** Salt and the phosphorus contained in sodas are both calcium-depleting minerals. If your diet is high in junk foods or you eat out several times a week you are probably consuming excessive amounts.

~ **Check your medications.** Several medications can increase the likelihood of bone loss. Among these are adrenal corticosteroids (cortisone-like drugs), anticoagulants (blood thinners), aluminum-containing antacids, some chemotherapy medications, antidepressants, certain diuretics, and some antibiotics. Check with your health care provider for possible side effects and how to counter them.

⌒ **Limit alcohol consumption.** Daily intake beyond a small glass of wine or beer can interfere with calcium absorption.

Sesame Seeds

The tiny sesame seed delivers a big nutritional boost toward growing healthy bones. This tasty seed is almost 19 percent protein and is richly endowed with B vitamins, calcium, and minerals. Try to find unhulled, whole sesame seeds; these are darker in color and considerably richer in nutrients than their white, hulled cousins.

A good way to add sesame seeds to your diet is to replace peanut butter with organic, crunchy sesame butter. I also like to make sweet sesame snack balls by combining sesame butter with enough whole sesame seeds to form a stiff paste. Add honey to sweeten, then form into small balls, and roll in unsweetened coconut shreds. Refrigerate, then enjoy. Yum!

- **Prevent falls.** Practice yoga or t'ai chi to improve balance, coordination, and flexibility.
- **Enjoy a little sun exposure.** I said a little, not a lot! Fifteen minutes a day of unprotected exposure to the sun's rays will aid in the development of vitamin D within the skin, which enhances calcium absorption in the intestines.

Stress-Busting Techniques

In these modern, fast-paced times, stress is unavoidable. During times of adversity, your reflexes naturally kick in and the adrenaline starts pumping. Heart rate, blood pressure, respiration, and blood sugar levels increase and muscles tense. The body's fight-or-flight mechanism is in high gear and the alarm is about to go off.

The highest reward for a man's toil is not what he gets for it, but what he becomes because of it.

—JOHN RUSKIN

Regain Control — and Your Cool

Before your stress alarm sounds and your world falls to pieces, learn to manage your stress and improve your health by following these tips. Always be proactive in making healthy lifestyle decisions.

Be realistic. You can't be everywhere at the same time, nor can you be all things to all people. Trying to be superhuman is a feat best left to Superman. Tackle the most important tasks first and the lesser priorities later. I begin my day by writing down all the tasks needing my attention and check them off one by one as the day goes by. This is very satisfying and gives me a sense of accomplishment.

Be aware. Learn to notice your body's specific stress signals. You can easily tell when your blood pressure is up: your palms can be sweaty, chest is tight, neck tense, stomach is in knots, or heart is pumping faster than normal. Other emotional and physical signs of stress might include difficulty concentrating, general irritability or annoyance, trembling, feeling "keyed up," insomnia or sleeping too much, feeling out of control or an urge to run and hide, finding yourself easily startled by small sounds, and feeling mental pressure from within yourself to be constantly productive.

Look forward to something. Plan a mini-vacation, go on a second honeymoon, take a day trip to a historical garden. When

There is nothing either good or bad, but thinking makes it so.

—WILLIAM SHAKESPEARE, *HAMLET*

stress strikes, recall the event you've planned for the near future and visualize the people you'll encounter and places you'll explore. Just looking forward to something enjoyable can instill a bit of tranquility.

~ **Learn to say no.** Eliminate activities that are not absolutely necessary in your life right now, learn to compromise, and by all means be flexible.

~ **Take a deep breath.** When the day isn't going your way, take a breather. Sit down and close your eyes. Press one finger over your right nostril and inhale deeply and slowly through your left. Exhale through your mouth. Now press one finger over your left nostril and repeat the procedure. Alternate this method 5 times on each side. Sure does the trick for me!

~ **Clear up the clutter.** A messy, unorganized home or office instantly stresses you upon entering. I know I'm not as productive when the trash can is overflowing, papers are in piles nearly falling from my desk, and the floor is littered with more piles.

~ **Get up, go outside, and blow off steam.** Take a brisk walk, ride your bicycle, or play a game of volleyball. The combination of exercise and fresh air will reduce tension, unclutter your mind, ease your frustration, improve your sleep, self-esteem, and well-being, and energize your mind and body. Not feeling energetic? Try a meditative yoga class instead.

~ **Relax with herbal tea.** Drink a cup or two daily of chamomile, catnip, passion-flower, skullcap, hops, or valerian tea. Pour a cup of boiling water over 1 or 2 teaspoons of dried herb, cover and steep for about 10 minutes. These mild-tasting herbs contain tranquilizing compounds traditionally known to ease stress without becoming addictive or making you feel groggy.

~ **Good nutrition makes a difference.** Be sure your diet includes the full complex of B vitamins — the antistress vitamins — and plenty of antioxidants (see Age-Defying Antioxidants, page 12). Limit the intake of caffeine and alcohol, which disturb sleep patterns, deplete your sources of vitamins C and B complex, and give you the jitters.

~ **Indulge in a stress-reducing massage.** By massaging the area immediately to either side of the spinal column the therapist can stimulate an acid toxin release from the tense muscles, resulting in simultaneous relaxation for the body and psyche. Ask for a massage combined with aromatherapy or an Ayurvedic scalp massage, if available.

~ **Laugh!** Laughter is physiologically stress relieving due to its ability to deepen breathing, oxygenate the blood, and ease muscle tension. I love watching a funny movie or listening to a comedian. It's a great way to relieve the tendency to worry and become anxious.

~ **"Don't worry, be happy."** Worrying is unproductive and fills your mind with unnecessary, time-consuming thoughts that limit your ability to enjoy living. Instead, focus on a project or hobby that gives you great satisfaction and takes your mind off your problems for awhile.

~ **Make a change for the better.** Do whatever it takes to erase or minimize the distress in your life. Unhappy at work? Look for a better, more fulfilling job. Fighting with your spouse? Seek counseling. Money too tight? Talk to a financial planner or design a budget. Lonely and depressed? Join a church, gym, or sign up for a new group hobby or activity.

⌐ Even one negative stress in your life can cause a serious health risk leading to loss of vitality and longevity. Whether your stress is financial, marital, work-related, lifestyle-related, or familial, talk to someone — don't keep all of your distress and worries to yourself. Explaining your feelings to a psychologist, psychiatrist, or minister may be of considerable assistance in putting your life back into perspective. Don't be ashamed if you feel out of control. Everyone needs a bit of sound, helpful advice now and again.

Develop "Mindfulness"

Every step you take is upon holy ground. Every moment is imbued with wonder and miracles.

— SUSAN SMITH JONES, CHOOSE RADIANT HEALTH & HAPPINESS

Mindfulness is the ability to live completely in the present, in the moment, focused on and aware of the here and now. Daily life provides plenty of opportunities to become more aware of both our inner life and our surroundings. "Like it or not, this moment is all we really have to work with," Jon Kabat-Zinn points out in *Wherever You Go, There You Are.* And as Joan Duncan Oliver acknowledges in *Contemplative Living,* "When we fall into daydreaming and automatic responses, we find ourselves anywhere but here."

Mindfulness is about moment-to-moment awareness instead of scattered awareness. Being mindful helps you group together the distracting bits of information demanding your attention and refocus on the now, the present. By simply allowing your attention to be fully focused on each moment you'll not fret about the future or look back on your life with a sense of regret.

Every day counts. Every hour counts. Every moment counts. Never let the small stuff pass you by. The small stuff makes the big picture brighter, deeper, and bolder! As the old saying goes, little things often mean the most.

Mindfulness-based stress reduction can cultivate relaxation, open the mind to greater insight, improve self-esteem, heal chronic illness, heal anxiety disorders, ease physical symptoms of pain, and enhance health and well-being. This type of stress reduction can include various forms of meditation and the practice of yoga. For information on teachers and classes in your area, contact local yoga studios, colleges, and universities and inquire about mindfulness-based stress reduction workshops.

Need More Sleep?

That's a foolish question — of course you do! Today's adult is tired. It's a plain and simple fact. We're pulled in too many directions, have far too many demands on our lives; something has to go in order just to keep up, and that something is usually our precious sleep. And when we do finally get to bed, many times we find that we're so keyed-up that sleep eludes us. Our minds race, engineering a strategy for coping with the next busy day.

When sleeping women wake, mountains move.

—CHINESE PROVERB

According to the National Sleep Foundation, though most experts recommend at least 8 hours of sleep per night, adults in the United States get significantly less. On average, working adults sleep only 6 hours and 54 minutes per weeknight, almost an hour less than they're due.

And further, when U.S. adults were asked to rank four strategies for maintaining good health — namely, getting enough sleep, managing stress, good nutrition, and regular exercise — sleep came in a lowly third! Say it isn't so! Receiving adequate sleep should become a priority for us all.

Insomnia is extremely common; up to one-third of the population suffers from it, some chronically. Sleep robbers include anxiety, disease, depression, stress, pain, hormonal changes, poor sleep habits, certain medical conditions (such as sleep apnea and restless leg syndrome), nontraditional working hours, and parenting young children.

As a whole, we are a sleep-deprived society, and it takes its toll on our looks, moods, and health. Sleep is critical to good health and well-being. It rejuvenates the mind, body, and spirit and enables you to function at peak capacity. Here are some tips for blissful sleep that I hope will have you feeling and looking fabulous in 40 winks.

~ **Create an optimal sleep environment.** This includes a mattress that offers ideal support and comfort; a dark room (see below); steady, soothing, low sounds like a whirring fan; and a room temperature of 60 to 65 degrees Fahrenheit, which is optimal for sleep.

~ **Increase productivity.** Most people shove sleep aside in favor of working more hours with the belief that they're maximizing efficiency, but in fact the opposite is true. You will be more creative, more expressive, and so much more efficient when your brain is alert and oxygenated.

~ **Relax before bedtime.** Find yourself too geared up to fall asleep at bedtime? Create a ritual for quality sleep. A cup of hot chamomile, catnip, or valerian (if you can stand the taste) tea works wonders. Hot milk with a dash of nutmeg or a cup of homemade, low-sugar hot cocoa are helpful for many people. You may want to take a soothing bath and soak in aromatherapeutic bubbles scented with lavender, Roman chamomile, or neroli essential oil.

~ **Eat several small meals throughout the day to stabilize your sugar level.** If you're hungry and hypoglycemic when it's time for bed, you will have trouble falling and staying asleep.

~ **Exercise vigorously in the morning.** By evening you'll be naturally tired. Vigorous exercise right before bedtime can be too stimulating for many people.

~ **Avoid hot, spicy foods at dinner, as well as caffeine or alcohol.**

Rest, rest,
perturbèd spirit.

—WILLIAM
SHAKESPEARE,
HAMLET

⁓ **Wear comfortable, preferably cotton, clothing to bed — or sleep au naturel.**

⁓ **Keep your bedroom as dark as possible to enhance melatonin production.** Melatonin is the hormone produced by the pineal gland that brings on drowsiness and sleep. Even small amounts of light entering your bedroom can interrupt its production, so pull the shades, turn off the television, and put the nightlight in the bathroom. If you must, wear a sleep mask.

⁓ **Go to bed by 10 P.M.** Generally, the more sleep you receive before midnight, the better you'll feel in the morning.

⁓ **Don't work or discuss work in the bedroom.** It's too distracting.

⁓ **Give yourself a nice foot or hand massage prior to sleep.** Even better, offer to give your significant other a brief massage if they'll return the favor.

⁓ **Once in bed, lie on your back, close your eyes, place your arms by your sides, and take long, deep, easy breaths through your nose; then slowly exhale through the mouth.** Let your mind focus only on your breathing. This exercise almost always lures me into a deep, sound sleep.

Boost Your Immunity

There is much talk today about immune system breakdown and the need to protect the immune system and maintain its strength and functioning. The term *immune* means to be protected from something harmful or disagreeable. This system is your first and often best line of defense against the onslaught of "foreign" invaders such as harmful bacteria, viruses, parasites, fungi, yeasts, germs, environmental chemicals, insect bites, foreign particles (such as splinters), or even a simple paper cut.

Your immune system works 24 hours a day largely unnoticed — that is, until something invades your body or the system fails. If a mosquito bites you, your skin swells, itches, and gets red. That's your immune system at work attempting to rid your body of the poison. A splinter may cause similar swelling, or even an infection.

When a harmful bacteria or virus enters your system and your immune system attempts to fight it off, a cold or flu may develop. Most harmful invaders are stopped in their tracks before they have a chance to take hold in your body, but if the immune system is weakened, all manner of problems can develop, such as bronchitis, pneumonia, chronic fatigue syndrome, mononucleosis, cancer, lupus, *Candida albicans*, herpes, staphylococcus and streptococcus infections, and arthritis.

With age, unfortunately, comes the increased risk of decreased immunity. Some common problems can include slowed wound healing; autoimmune disorders such as multiple sclerosis, Graves disease, diabetes mellitus, and rheumatoid arthritis; increased infection risk; and cancer.

The key to boosting your immune system is simple. Give it what it needs by feeding it the appropriate fuels: organic, whole foods, immune boosting herbs, purified water, fresh air, and exercise. Be sure to balance work with rest, maintain a zest for living, control your stress level, engage in a soul-satisfying spiritual practice, and maintain loving relationships.

The Herbal Immune Tincture on page 68 can help enhance your immune system when its help is most needed.

Look to your health; and if you have it . . . value it next to a good conscience; for health is the second blessing that we mortals are capable of; a blessing that money cannot buy.

— IZAAC WALTON,
THE COMPLEAT
ANGLER

Herbal Immune Tincture

This herbal formula is designed to enhance immune system functioning and boost memory and mental awareness, and is simple to make. All herbs are in dried form.

1 sterilized quart canning jar with lid

3 tablespoons osha root *(Ligusticum porteri)*

2 tablespoons St.-John's-wort *(Hypericum perforatum)*

1 tablespoon Siberian ginseng root *(Eleutherococcus senticosus)*

3 tablespoons echinacea root *(Echinacea angustifolia)*

2 tablespoons astragalus root *(Astragalus membranaceus)*

1 teaspoon peppermint leaves *(Mentha piperita)*

1 teaspoon gotu kola leaves *(Centella asiatica)*

1 teaspoon ginkgo leaves *(Ginkgo biloba)*

1 small yellow onion, minced

20 garlic cloves, minced

⅛ teaspoon cayenne powder or ¼ teaspoon flakes

1 large bottle of 80-proof vodka
(an inexpensive brand is fine)
1 5" x 5" square of plastic film or
plastic sandwich baggie

1. On the evening of the full moon, add
   all herbs and vegetables to a quart jar.
   Pour vodka to within 1 inch of the top.
2. Place plastic wrap or a plastic baggie
   over the top of the jar and then screw
   on the metal lid. (The plastic prevents
   the metal from rusting.) Shake daily
   and store in a dark, dry, cool place.
   Allow formula to synergize for at least
   8 weeks, and up to 6 months for maximum potency.
3. On the evening prior to the full moon,
   strain mixture through a strainer lined
   with pantyhose (so that all fine partic-
   ulate matter is caught). Press herbs
   with the back of a large spoon or with
   your fingers in order to extract all of
   the liquid.
4. Divide the liquid into several 2-ounce,
   dropper-top, dark glass bottles. Store
   the bottles on a dark, cool, dry shelf
   until ready to use. Your tincture should
   last for many years.

5. To use, take 1–2 droppersful daily directly on the tongue or diluted in a cup of water. Can be taken year round, but I generally recommend six days on with the seventh day off. Repeat for one month, then take the next month off. Then begin the cycle again.

Yield: Approximately 2–3 cups

Digest with Ease

The adage "You are what you eat" should actually be, "You are what you properly digest, assimilate, and eliminate." No matter how healthy your diet, if you can't properly digest your food, then you can't assimilate the necessary nutrients to keep your body functioning at optimal levels.

Your digestive system consists of a 25 to 35 foot long, winding, twisting tube that receives food at one end (the mouth) and eliminates the spent product from the other end (the anus).

Indigestion is a major problem incurred by a large percentage of the population, especially the over-40 crowd. The manufacturers of popular antacids are quite aware of this dilemma and are quick to capitalize on America's discomfort. Just turn on the television and their ads instantly appear right after lunch and dinnertime. They offer quick, though temporary, relief to those who regularly gorge themselves on massive quantities of greasy, spicy, or fiberless foods, or those who lead stress-filled lives, smoke, drink alcohol on a regular basis, and eat on the run. If you continually stuff yourself past the exploding point, eat too fast or under stressful conditions, or make poor food and lifestyle choices, your body is bound to rebel.

Disorderly Conduct

Digestive disorders left untreated can eventually lead to serious problems, such as cirrhosis of the liver, jaundice, hepatitis, diverticular disease, and cancers of the digestive system. Anyone suffering from digestive problems can attest to how unbearable the disease makes everyday life.

Repeatedly reaching for a commercial antacid is not the answer to digestive problems. The answer lies in simply observing the rules of civilized eating and allowing your body's chemistry to do what it's designed to do, ensuring complete, comfortable digestion.

~ **Always sit when eating.** When I'm super busy, I find that I often eat while standing and trying to do other chores. This makes for an unsatisfying meal and frequently ends in severe indigestion. I notice a big difference in the way I feel if I simply take 20 minutes to sit down, relax, and enjoy my meal.

~ **Say grace.** Offer a few words of reverence or have a moment of silence for the nourishment you are about to consume. This simple act alone causes you to pause before eating, thereby putting your digestive system at ease.

~ **Give yourself an enzymatic boost.** I find that when I suffer from an occasional bout of indigestion, a couple of plant-based enzyme capsules taken right after my meal really do the trick. Available in health food stores, they assist the digestive system naturally without disrupting the acid/alkaline balance.

~ **Eat raw veggies.** Begin your meals with a raw vegetable salad or glass of freshly made raw vegetable juice, such as a carrot, celery, and apple blend. Chew or sip slowly. Raw foods, which happen to be severely lacking in the American diet today, are chock-full of live enzymes that aid in the digestive process. As a bonus, you'll tend to eat less if you fill up on a large, fiber-rich salad first!

~ **Eat in a quiet atmosphere.** Turn off the television, put away the newspaper, and eliminate other distractions.

~ **Heed nature's call.** Make time to go to the bathroom. By all means, don't hold it all in — you'll just be miserable. Regularity is one of the keys to a happy, proper functioning digestive system.

~ **Chew, chew, chew!** Digestion begins in the mouth. Chew each bite until it is nearly liquefied, then swallow. That way the enzymes present in your saliva have a chance to initiate the digestive process.

Thorough chewing also promotes slower food consumption.

~ **Don't eat when angry, stressed-out, or physically exhausted.** Digestive juices are suppressed during emotionally or physically demanding times. Digestion requires lots of energy. Wait until you are relaxed and calm before you eat.

~ **Don't drink lots of fluids during your meal.** Sipping is okay. A stomach full of liquids slows the digestion of solid foods and dilutes the digestive juices. Also, avoid ice-cold beverages; they interfere with digestion.

~ **Try to eat at approximately the same times each day.** Your digestive system likes a regular schedule.

~ **Don't gulp your food.** Eating behavior that mimics Rover's can cause you to swallow air, resulting in belching.

~ **Leave the table** when you think you could still stomach a little bit more. It takes your brain up to 30 minutes to register that it is full.

Love Your Liver

Your liver, located on the right side under your lower ribs, is the most metabolically complex organ in the entire body. Explains Dr. Richard Schulze in the May 2000 issue of his bimonthly newsletter *Get Well!*, the liver "Detoxifies, metabolizes, renders harmless and eliminates harmful toxic poisons, chemicals, and substances from your blood. It produces many different enzymes that actually convert toxic poisons into harmless chemicals and then they are eliminated in the bile that your liver excretes."

Your liver does so much for your body that I'd need an entire book to explain all of its functions, but suffice to say it is vital that you keep it healthy for good digestion. To encourage liver health, eat a nutritious diet consisting of mostly whole, organic, high-fiber foods and plenty of purified water. Avoid junk foods, alcohol, fatty and fried foods, processed and chemical-laden foods, smoking, and drugs. Remember, a sluggish, clogged liver, produces a sluggish, unhealthy, lethargic you!

Don Ollsin, herbalist and author of *Herbal Healing Journey*, suggests organic dandelion root tea and diluted lemon water as daily tonics for the liver. The lemon water is important for its natural hydrochloric

To eat is human; to digest, divine.

—CHARLES T. COPELAND

acid that the liver converts into some 6 billion different enzymes. Dandelion root and leaves are first class liver cleansers and tonics. Dandelion provides a rich source of easily-absorbable minerals, clears congestion of the spleen, gallbladder, pancreas, bladder, and kidneys, and is rich in organic sodium being of tremendous benefit to the stomach and intestines.

Heart Disease: Are You at Risk?

According to the American Heart Association, cardiovascular disease is America's number one killer. It claims the lives of 41 percent of the more than 2.3 million Americans who die each year. Almost 60 million Americans have some form of cardiovascular disease, ranging from congenital heart defects to high blood pressure and hardening of the arteries.

Exactly how and why heart disease originates in the body is a difficult, complex, and often confusing question to answer. You can reduce your risk of heart disease by becoming aware of your risk factors —

personal lifestyle habits and genetic traits that can make you more or less prone to develop a particular disease. Risk factors such as age, family history, and sex are beyond your control. The major risk factors over which you can exert considerable control are tobacco smoking, high cholesterol levels, high blood pressure, physical inactivity, and obesity.

4 Steps to a Healthy Heart

Reducing lifestyle-related risks yields a big payoff towards preventing heart disease. Follow these four rules:

1. **Don't smoke.** Did you know that smoking is the single most preventable cause of death in the United States and that the risk of heart attack is more than twice that of nonsmokers? Smokers, when they do have an attack, are more likely to die and die suddenly than are nonsmokers. Second-hand smoke in your environment also significantly increases your risk for heart disease. The good news is that when you do quit smoking, regardless of how long you smoked, your risk of heart disease makes a rapid and dramatic drop.

2. **Exercise.** Any type of moderate to vigorous physical exercise, preferably a type you enjoy, should be done at least 30 minutes per day. Yoga, stretching, and weight lifting are terrific as supplemental exercises, but you still need to get your heart pounding for a sustained period of time in order to burn fat and strengthen the heart muscle and surrounding tissues and arteries.

3. **Stay slim.** Overweight is defined as a body mass index (BMI) of 25.0 to less than 30.0. Being within this range puts you at moderate risk for heart disease. A BMI of 30.0 and higher (30 pounds or more overweight) is classified as obese and puts you at high risk. To calculate your exact BMI number, multiply your weight in pounds by 705, divide by your height in inches, then divide again by your height in inches. Note that some athletes and body builders with dense muscle mass may have a high BMI but very little body fat.

4. **Eat a heart-healthy diet.** Food should be nutritious as well as pleasurable to the taste buds. It is not necessary to eat only lettuce, sprout, and tofu sandwiches on a slab or flavorless bran bread in order to keep

your heart healthy. See chapter 1 for tasty dietary suggestions.

Preventive Health Measures: Screening Tests

Quite often, especially if you're under 50 years of age and feeling robust and healthy, the thought of scheduling a visit to your health practitioner for a routine screening test is dismissed as unnecessary. But routine physicals for healthy people quite often include a screening test or two that can spot potential diseases at an early, yet still curable stage prior to any noticeable occurrence of symptoms. Screening tests can also rule out a disease for which you are potentially at risk, either due to family medical history or exposure to outside influences.

How often should you have the various health screenings performed? There are general frequency rules to follow, but your health-care practitioner should make individualized recommendations based on your present health, family medical history, and other outside factors (such as prescription medication intake, involvement with recreational drugs, exposure to workplace chemicals, and smoking habits).

The following is a chart of periodic medical tests you should have even when you are in perfect health. These guidelines are based largely on recommendations by the American Cancer Society and U.S. Preventive Services Task Force.

~ **Blood pressure:** Every 2 years after age 18 if reading is normal, or as recommended by health practitioner.

~ **Bone density scan (dual energy x-ray absorptiometry, or DEXA):** A scan of spinal, hip, and forearm bone density at first sign of menopause or earlier if there is a family history of osteoporosis, past history of broken bones, past or present intake of prescription corticosteroids, or history of hyperthyroidism or hyperparathyroidism.

~ **Dental checkup:** Annually.

~ **Eye exam:** Every 3 to 5 years, and more often after age 50.

~ **Cholesterol test (serum lipid profile):** Once while in 20s, then at least every 5 years or as recommended.

~ **Digital rectal exam:** 50 years old or earlier if at risk.

~ **Fecal occult blood test (FOBT):** Every 1 to 2 years after age 50.

~ **Colonoscopy:** Every 5 to 10 years after age 50.

~ **Flexible sigmoidoscopy:** Every 3 to 5 years after age 50.

~ **Mammogram:** Baseline mammogram between ages 35 and 39, then a regular mammogram every 2 years between ages 40 and 49, and then annually from age 50 on.

~ **Clinical breast exam:** Every 3 years starting at age 20 and annually after age 40.

~ **Breast self-exam:** Monthly.

~ **Pap test or smear:** Annually after age 18.

~ **Pelvic exam:** Annually after age 18.

~ **Skin cancer check:** Preferably by a dermatologist; annually after 50 or earlier if at risk.

~ **Skin self-exam:** Monthly.

Reiki: Hands-on Healing

Reiki, pronounced (RAY-kee), is a traditional art of physical, emotional, and spiritual healing that draws its name from the Japanese characters *rei,* meaning spirit or

God-consciousness, and *ki* meaning life-force energy. This form of energetic healing bases its theory on ancient Tibetan healing techniques that were rediscovered in the mid-1800s by Dr. Mikao Usui, a Japanese Buddhist.

Reiki operates on the theory that the universal life energy, which permeates all living things, can be channeled through the body via the natural energy pathways — the chakras, nadis, and meridians — and the aura surrounding the body. This channeling releases any energy blockages, allowing the natural life force to increase or balance. The result is enhanced well-being.

What to Expect

During a typical 60 to 90 minute healing session, the reiki practitioner will have you lie on your back, fully clothed, on a massage-type table. Next she will place her hands, palms down, in different positions over the body and hold each position for 3 to 5 minutes. During this time, you draw in whatever energy you need from the universe. The practitioner is believed to amplify this energy by placing her hands on your body.

Unlike massage, the touch is very gentle with little or no pressure. If you prefer, reiki can be performed without touching. The practitioner simply places her hands a few inches above your body in the areas she would normally touch. During the session some people report feeling heat, tingling sensations, or seeing colors.

Reiki is a very gentle form of healing, yet can have powerful results. It is beneficial for a variety of health problems, from stress reduction to cuts and bruises, from headaches to low self-esteem, from heart disease to cancer. You don't have to be sick to appreciate reiki; it benefits people of all ages and can do no harm to anyone.

What did I receive from my two reiki sessions? I had my first session in 1998 while in the midst of a personal crisis. During the session, I felt a sense of complete peace. My body felt very heavy, as if in a deep meditative state. Toward the end I began to feel shaky and weepy. In fact, I cried on and off for the next two days. It was an incredible release for me. A few months later I had another session, and I talked the entire time. I felt light and energetic afterward.

Two sessions, same practitioner, same techniques, but totally different outcomes. I received what I needed each time.

Can Anyone Learn Reiki?

Yes, anyone can learn to give reiki to themselves as well as others. There are three degrees of reiki, each requiring an attunement or ritual in which the reiki master attunes you, or opens you to the reiki energy, so that you can become an energy channel. Upon receiving the third degree of reiki, you become a reiki master. At this point you are able to educate others and do reiki attunements.

To find a practitioner or reiki master in your area, check out the advertising section of your local alternative healing magazine. Health-food store bulletin boards are a good source, as is word of mouth. Many practitioners do not advertise, but they feel that if a person is sincere in her desire to learn or benefit from reiki, she will find the appropriate master.

3

Revitalize with Exercise

Simple daily exercise is key to living life to the fullest. Exercise can be as simple as walking the dog, cleaning the house, or gardening, or as vigorous as rollerblading, downhill skiing, and marathon running. The choice is yours.

Exercising for at least 30 minutes a day, 5 days per week, will help slow the aging process, increase your metabolism, increase bone and muscle mass, improve range of motion and general mobility, improve balance and coordination, improve sleep patterns and immune function, and reduce the risk of disease. Your skin will take on a luminescence that comes with increased circulation to the extremities. You'll feel calmer, more alert, and more confident. Find an activity you enjoy and do it every day to help ensure a lifetime of good health.

Yoga, T'ai Chi, and Qi Gong: Ancient Teachings for Modern Times

We Westerners have much to learn from older civilizations. Until recently, most forms of exercise practiced on this side of the globe have focused primarily on the physical aspects and benefits of exercise: cardiovascular improvement, increased strength and stamina, weight loss, and toning. Yoga, ta'i chi, and qi gong emphasize the physical, but they round out the exercise experience by also focusing on the mental and spiritual aspects of well-being.

Why Do Yoga?

Yoga is a system of exercise and meditation developed in India more than 5,000 years ago that is still evolving today. In Sanskrit, the classical language of India, yoga means a method of uniting — a union of body, mind, and spirit. Studying and practicing yoga require your efforts in all three aspects in order to heal or unify the whole.

Yoga, a gentle, slow-moving exercise, draws awareness inward instead of focusing merely on the physical. It uses *asanas* — poses or postures — to work muscles. During the postures, you remain in the present by concentrating on movement and breathing, thus creating the awareness necessary to become in tune with your body.

Is Yoga for Me?

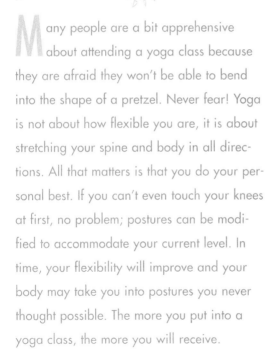

Many people are a bit apprehensive about attending a yoga class because they are afraid they won't be able to bend into the shape of a pretzel. Never fear! Yoga is not about how flexible you are, it is about stretching your spine and body in all directions. All that matters is that you do your personal best. If you can't even touch your knees at first, no problem; postures can be modified to accommodate your current level. In time, your flexibility will improve and your body may take you into postures you never thought possible. The more you put into a yoga class, the more you will receive.

Yoga brings into balance your body, mind, and spirit.

Practicing yoga is a perfect way to help deal with the Western cultural problems of incorrect posture, aggressive lifestyles, job stress, demanding family lives, overeating and indigestion, and stiff muscles and joints. The many benefits of yoga include increased flexibility, profound relaxation, clarity of thought, and increased muscle tone and strength, as well as improved balance, coordination, concentration, and oxygen intake. Yoga practice can also help manage anxiety, arthritis, asthma, back pain, blood pressure, carpal tunnel syndrome, chronic fatigue, depression, diabetes, heart disease, menopausal symptoms, migraines, multiple sclerosis, and osteoporosis.

Hatha yoga is the most popular style of yoga practiced in the Western world. It is less meditative and tends to be more physical, incorporating strength, stretching, and breathing. Still, there are many styles of yoga, and they differ from teacher to teacher and from one organization or teaching philosophy to another. You may encounter the style names Iyengar, Kripalu,

Kundalini, Sivananda, Ashtanga, Bikram, and many others. Try a few different classes until you find a style that suits your lifestyle.

Qi Gong

Qi gong or *ch'i kung* (pronounced CHEE-GUNG) means to work with one's *qi*. It is an ancient Taoist healing system that is similar to yoga in that it emphasizes proper breathing, meditation, and specific body movements to stimulate or open and direct the free flow of qi throughout the body. The main objective of qi gong is to balance the *yang*, or "masculine," active energy with the *yin*, or "feminine," receptive energy. It seeks to harmonize human nature with spiritual nature through two forms of practice: still practice and moving practice.

This meditative form of healing art can both energize and relax your body. It has been linked with some powerful health benefits, such as increased oxygen intake and usage, lowered blood pressure, increased levels of calming and soothing endorphins and serotonin in the brain, and a vigorous immune system.

Circulate Your Qi

According to Traditional Chinese Medicine (TCM), *qi* (also spelled *chi*) is life energy or the fundamental activating, ever-changing force of life. It is expressed in vastly different forms in nature, the physical body, the mineral kingdom, and the plant kingdom, yet it unifies the physical, mental, and spiritual qualities of energy throughout the universe.

Methods for increasing the circulation of qi throughout the body and mind include yoga, all types of dance, sports, moderate aerobic exercise, t'ai chi, qi gong, playing, and laughing. Breathing exercises and meditation also strengthen qi.

T'ai Chi

T'ai chi (pronounced TIE CHEE), meaning "the way of the fist," is a martial art form that grew out of *qi gong*. In China, whether in large corporate exercise rooms, city parks, or local green spaces, you can see hundreds of people practicing this ancient art form early in the morning. The long form consists of a sequence of 100 or more different movements performed in coordination with breathing in a slow, deliberate, ritualized, graceful manner that flows gently from one movement to the next. The short form consists of 24 sequential movements. T'ai chi is a powerful form of physical, mental, and spiritual exercise that tones and stretches the body, improving flexibility, strength, and control while harmonizing and strengthening the mind/body connection. It is particularly useful for managing stress and tension.

T'ai chi's gentle continuity of movement allows the body to relax while increasing circulation and qi, thus enhancing vitality throughout the body. Anyone — whether a sedentary couch potato or seasoned athlete — can practice this martial art. Initially, a qualified instructor is recommended to learn proper form, breathing, and posture, but a good book or video can also be valuable guides. Ta'i chi and qi gong classes are offered in *dojos*, or practice halls, and sometimes in health clubs.

Having an Energy Crisis?

Did you know that fatigue is the number one complaint heard by today's health-care practitioners? I'm not surprised! Energy deficits can stem from a variety of sources: insufficient sleep, poor diet, illness, infection, some medications, emotional stressors, lack of exercise, or simply working too much with no down time for fun.

Life is a daring adventure or nothing.

—HELEN KELLER

All Aboard the Energy Express

Here are a handful of strategies to boost your motivation and keep your engine running smoothly and efficiently. If you still feel tired after trying these tips, consult your physician or health-care practitioner.

⁓ **Eat more protein.** Keep a diet diary for a week. Write down everything you put in your mouth. Is your protein intake less than 20 to 30 percent of your daily calories? If so, you could be consuming inadequate quantities of this essential nutrient. Add a few servings of eggs, lean poultry, beef, wild game, fish, whole grains, or beans to your weekly menu. If you're a highly active person, you may need to eat a little bit more protein than your more sedentary peers. Consult a nutritionist or good nutrition book for more information.

〜 **Take a whiff.** For an aromatherapeutic energy boost, keep a bottle of stimulating essential oil handy. Place a couple of drops onto a tissue and inhale deeply for a few minutes. Good essential oils to try are peppermint, cypress, *Eucalyptus globulus* or *Eucalyptus radiata*, and geranium.

〜 **Drink up.** Your brain is more than 70 percent water by weight, and if this level drops too low you'll feel headachy, tired, and "foggy." So heed the tried-and-true recommendation: 8 glasses of purified water daily, more if you're active or it's hot or the humidity is low.

〜 **Take a hike.** Or a walk. Or march in place. Climb a few sets of stairs. Just get physical. Any type of aerobic exercise, performed for just 5 minutes, will increase circulation and oxygen flow throughout your body, thus boosting energy levels.

〜 **Manage your stress.** The daily stresses of work, family, and life in general all impact your health and drain your energy.

Dream as if you'll live forever. Live as if you'll die today.

—JAMES DEAN

Learn to deal with, control, or eliminate many of the stressors that are dragging you down. See Stress-Busting Techniques on page 55 for ideas.

~ **Have a light lunch.** Loading up at lunchtime can leave you feeling drowsy or light-headed, especially if you've eaten a carbohydrate-heavy meal, such as pasta, rice and beans, or garlic bread. Instead, opt for a light- to moderate-sized meal with approximately 500 to 800 calories, and be sure to include a portion of protein along with those carbohydrates to promote that clear-headed, alert feeling.

~ **Pep up with peppermint.** When in need of an instant lift, drink a cup of strong, iced peppermint tea. The coldness will shock your system into alertness and the peppermint flavor and aroma will stimulate your senses. Additionally, keep a small spray bottle filled with peppermint tea in the refrigerator so you can spritz your face when you need a quick boost.

~ **Hit the hay.** Inadequate sleep will leave the healthiest people dragging their heels. Sooner or later you'll pay the price with how you feel, think, and look. I tell my skin-care clients that sleep is the best-kept beauty and energy secret around.

⌒ **Have your blood tested.** Pernicious anemia (vitamin B_{12} deficiency), iron-deficiency anemia, or a folic acid, biotin, vitamin B_2, or B_6 deficiency can lead to a less-than-optimal amount of oxygen being transported through your blood stream. These deficiencies can leave you feeling draggy and lethargic. Even if you think you're eating a healthy diet, you may not be getting enough of these essential nutrients, especially if you're a vegan or a menstruating woman. If you test positive for a deficiency, follow your doctor's orders by adjusting your diet accordingly. Your energy should soon return.

⌒ **Soak up some rays.** Natural light influences the level of melatonin, a brain hormone produced by the pineal gland, which regulates how sleepy you feel. Try to get 10 to 15 minutes — before 10:30 A.M. or after 4:30 P.M. — of unprotected sun exposure daily on your face, hands, arms, or legs.

⌒ **Focus on the positive.** A positive attitude is refreshing, rejuvenating, and makes you feel consistently upbeat. It's also contagious to those around you. On the contrary, negative emotions can really drain your enthusiasm and zest for life.

~ **Enjoy a cup of green tea.** This earthy-tasting, antioxidant-rich Asian tea has only one-fifth of the caffeine of black tea, so it shouldn't give you the shakes.

Live to a Ripe Old Age

"Do everything in moderation and go to church and you'll live to be an old-timer like me," says my 90-year-old grandfather. He eats a little of everything, doesn't smoke, maintains a large garden and a couple of beehives, and tends his small herd of cattle. His longevity secrets? He stays active, wears a quality sunscreen, loves his wife of 60-plus years, and loves God. He's slowed down a bit in recent years, but he's still quite energetic and agile for a man his age. Daily naps help keep his energy up, too.

Walk for Life

Remember Sir Isaac Newton's First Law of Motion? It states, "An object at rest tends to remain at rest. An object in motion tends to remain in motion." So how does this physics law relate to you? Well, try thinking of it this way: A sedentary body has no get-up-and-go and can easily remain sedentary, but an active body often has an easier time continuing to exercise throughout life because of increased energy and vitality. The less you do, the less you can do. The more you do, the more you can do. Energy begets energy. Get it?

What exercise do I, and thousands of health and fitness experts, recommend to recharge your life and get the fitness ball in motion? Walking. Brisk walking, in particular, is superior in many aspects to running and jogging in terms of overall health benefits. Why? First, almost everyone can walk. Second, your risk of injury is far less than for most other types of aerobic exercises. Third, you can do it almost anywhere. Finally, it's low cost; the only equipment required is a good pair of walking shoes.

Be not afraid of going slowly; be afraid only of standing still.

—CHINESE PROVERB

Burn, Baby, Burn

Want to get the most caloric bang out of your daily exercise time? The following exercises, which burn the most calories for time spent exercising, are based on the energy a 150-pound person would expend in one hour.

⁓ **Cross-country skiing.** One of the best exercises for overall body toning, skiing at a 5 mile per hour pace, which is quite vigorous, burns approximately 700 calories per hour.

⁓ **Snow shoveling.** Try throwing away your snow blower and picking up a shovel. This exercise, performed at a moderate pace, burns approximately 600 calories an hour. *Caution:* Snow shoveling can be extremely demanding for arm and back muscles. Pace yourself!

⁓ **Rollerblading.** This exercise will chisel the saddlebags off your hips and thighs in no time and give your heart a terrific workout. At a moderate skating pace, this activity burns approximately 600 calories per hour.

Mowing your lawn. Using a push mower versus a power mower provides all-over body conditioning and burns approximately 450 calories per hour.

Running. Running at a moderate pace, 5.5 miles per hour, burns approximately 650 calories per hour.

Walking. Speed walking at a 4 mile per hour pace works up a sweat and burns approximately 400 calories per hour.

Bicycling. Pumping those pedals at a moderate 10 mile per hour pace burns approximately 400 calories per hour.

Domestic Goddess work. This includes washing floors and windows, vacuuming, washing the car, ironing, hanging clothes out to dry, cleaning the bathroom, and other chores, and it burns approximately 250 calories per hour.

Weight lifting. Builds metabolism-boosting muscles and lifts and tones every muscle in your body. An hour of weight training burns approximately 300 calories.

Personally, I think walking is the best exercise for women. Running, jogging, jumping rope, and some vigorous aerobic activities can be extremely jarring and damaging to the joints and breasts. But walking is one exercise you can truly start ultra-slowly and gradually build up to speed.

Walking is convenient, plain and simple. You can walk around the block, in the mall, in the park, down a city street, by the ocean, in the woods, or on your treadmill in front of the television or while listening to music or books on tape. Just be sure that your chosen location is a safe one.

Walking Benefits for All Ages

A walking program will help prepare you for or protect you from all manner of health concerns, such as osteoporosis, weight gain, problem pregnancies, menopause, stress, muscle loss, flagging energy, heart disease, and stroke. Daily walking will go a long way toward keeping you happy and healthy. It fully engages your body, mind, and spirit.

~ **Put in your time.** Forty-five to sixty minutes daily: That's what your eventual goal should be. Sound like a long time? Well once you get started it's over in a flash, and, besides that, it's the amount of time necessary to spur your metabolism into burning plenty of fat and calories and give your heart a good workout.

Note: If you're a beginner or have been sedentary for a while, start a walking program slowly, doing what you can without too much stress on your body. As you get stronger, increase your intensity gradually.

⁓ **Go for the glow.** Brisk walking makes you sweat, and with this increased perspiration toxins are excreted through the skin. Within a few weeks after starting a walking program you'll definitely notice a more radiant, more clarified complexion.

⁓ **Pump those arms.** Don't just let your arms hang down by your sides as you walk, really swing and pump them. In addition to burning more calories and enabling you to walk faster, pumping will firm the pectoral muscles in your chest, giving the chest a more sculpted, rounded appearance.

⁓ **A pelvic plus.** With age (and childbirth) comes the tendency toward urinary incontinence. Walking will help to tighten the ligaments and muscles in the pelvic floor.

Make sure to do your Kegel exercises or pelvic diaphragm contractions daily, as well.

~ **Walking meditation.** Your mind can be totally relaxed and void of all thought or clearly focused on a particular idea while you move along. I frequently carry a little tape recorder or small pen and pad with me to jot down notes. Walking can also be a time of spiritual renewal.

~ **Mind your mood.** Walking will improve your outlook on life, lift depression, and boost your self-esteem and confidence. The exercise-induced beta-endorphins that the brain releases during exercise will help lessen mood swings and bouts of anxiety.

~ **Offset estrogen loss.** With menopause comes the loss of heart-protecting estrogen, increasing your risk of cardiovascular disease. Regular walking can raise good cholesterol (HDL) and lower bad cholesterol (LDL), lessening the risk of disease.

Improve Your Bottom Line

Does the nature of your daily work require that you sit down for long periods of time? If so, those hours spent sitting relatively motionless day after day limits the circulation to your backside and adds to the gradual spreading and flattening of your muscle tissue. Even if you don't sit down all day, simply by virtue of being a woman you're naturally "blessed" with a high percentage of body fat in this lower region, and you may have found that no matter how hard you work out, you're still not satisfied with your rear view.

Uphill Walking

Brisk, uphill walking, for a sustained period of time, especially as part of your daily walking routine, can actually give you a better overall workout than jogging, running, or going to the gym for an aerobics class. Walking uphill is your best bet for aerobic fat burning and anaerobic muscle conditioning. This activity will trim and tone your lower body, especially your posterior, in no time flat!

Techniques to Tone Your Tush

The following activities will strengthen and sculpt the muscles of your legs in addition to firming your gluteus maximus (the large muscle of the buttocks).

~ **Isometric squeezes.** These can be performed anywhere and no one else will even know you're doing them. Simply squeeze your buttocks as hard as you can, hold for 5 seconds, release. Repeat as many times as you can, as often as you can, throughout the day. This really revs up the posterior circulation.

~ **Perform forward or backward lunges, great exercises for lifting the derriere.** Make sure to keep the bent leg at a 90-degree angle with the knee directly over the ankle. The knee of the straight leg should be just a few inches off the floor — if you're able.

~ **Kick up your legs.** You don't have to be a Las Vegas showgirl to have long, lean legs and a tight butt. Place your left hand on a sturdy chair, stand straight and tall, and kick your right leg as high as you possibly can without slouching and bending at the waist. Do 10 kicks, then change legs. Work up to 100 kicks per leg daily.

~ **Reverse leg kick-backs.** Place your left hand on a sturdy chair and stand straight and tall. Now slowly lift your right leg behind you, with toe pointed, as high as you can; release, and repeat 10 times. Try not to bend or arch your back. Change legs. Work up to 100 kick-backs with each leg daily.

~ **Squats.** Stand with toes facing straight ahead, arms held straight out in front of you, and feet shoulder-width apart. Squat as if you are going to sit in a chair. When knees are bent at a 90-degree angle, clench your buttocks as hard as you can and return to a standing position. Release. Repeat 10 times. Work up to 50 squats, if possible.

~ **Climb the stairs.** Whether on a stair-stepping machine at the gym or climbing the stairs at work, this is one of the best exercises for complete leg and fanny toning. Gives your heart a great workout, too.

~ **Do step aerobics.** Similar to climbing stairs, step aerobics combines cardiovascular conditioning and an upper body workout while completely resculpting your lower body. A major calorie burner!

∼ **Walk on a treadmill set to a steep incline.** For maximum tush toning, lower the speed and increase the incline to the steepest you can comfortably handle and walk for as long as possible. You'll be amazed at the added lift your derriere receives. Don't be surprised if your legs are quite sore for a while afterward.

∼ **Pop in an exercise video that specifically targets this area.** There are many on the market and some take no more than fifteen minutes to perform. Just seeing the slim, firm instructor is enough motivation to stick with it.

Stay Motivated

You know exercise is good for you, but sometimes you're just not in the mood to move. The sofa looks more inviting, the television more interesting, and that batch of freshly made chocolate-pecan chunk cookies more enticing. These motivational tips will help get you off your spreading fanny and out running, walking, or gardening. Then you can enjoy a cookie — or two or three — guilt-free!

Let's Get Moving

When it comes to exercise, if you lack motivation, it's difficult to follow through. Use these strategies to make your daily workouts more appealing.

~ **Burn it and earn it.** Want a big piece of your favorite dessert? You'll have to walk about 4 miles to burn 400 calories, which is equal to a big wedge of pie or cake, large candy bar, or shake.

~ **Exercise first thing in the morning.** If you make early-morning exercise a daily habit, then there's no chance it can get shoved by the wayside later in the day.

~ **Reward yourself.** As a teen, my father used to pay me a dollar for every mile I ran as incentive to stay with my training program. You can adopt a similar program. Simply put a dollar or two into a jar each and every time you exercise. If you're consistent, soon you'll have enough money to buy that new smaller size outfit you've been wanting, or a new garden tool or golf club. Customize your incentive program and keep your eyes on the prize.

~ **Make exercise fun.** Rollerblade rather than walk if that's more exciting to

You just can't beat the person who never gives up.

— George "Babe" Ruth

you. Jump rope or play volleyball if that's your cup of tea. Exercise shouldn't be just another daily chore. If you look forward to having 30 to 60 minutes of active enjoyment each day, you're more apt to stick to your program.

~ **Train for a local 5k or 10k run or walk in your community**. Last spring, for three days each week, one of my friends and I trained for a 4-mile fun run to benefit a local library. It was our first competition ever and we loved it. We didn't break any speed records, but the camaraderie was exhilarating.

~ **Keep an exercise diary.** Each day, record how you feel, how your clothes fit, your energy level, bowel habits, condition of your skin, your mood, and stress level. As the weeks go by, you should begin to see a measurable improvement in quite a few of these personal markers.

~ **Add years to your life and life to your years.** Exercise will give you physical strength, boost endurance, and enhance health, enabling you to do all the things you long to do — for life! What more motivation do you need?

Throw Away the Remote Control

The United States is one of the fattest nations on earth. What's really shocking is that, today, nearly 25 percent of our young people are considered obese. This disturbing trend shows no sign of slowing, so it's critical that as a nation — for our sake and for the sake of our children — we take this issue seriously. Obesity does not merely affect appearance; it is often accompanied by heart problems, diabetes, liver problems, disorders of the connective tissues, back problems, and emotional issues.

Once a nation of slim people, powered by manual labor, we now rely heavily on machines for even the smallest of tasks. The calories once expended during daily activities are currently being collected on our thighs, posteriors, and stomachs. Instead of pushing a button for this and another for that, make an effort to do things the old-fashioned way for a change. You'll save exorbitant gymnasium membership fees and get a lot more accomplished in the meantime. You'll feel better, too.

Small Changes, Big Results

imple lifestyle choices can have a big impact on your health. Choose to be more active, and you'll feel better!

⌒ **Use a push lawn mower instead of a self-propelled one.** Afterward you'll feel as if you've had a complete workout.

⌒ **Split some wood.** Have a fireplace? Then call your local wood supplier and have him deliver 18" log sections instead of pre-split wood and split it yourself. My grandfather always says, "Wood should warm you twice: once when you split and stack it, and then again when you burn it." Log sections are much less expensive than pre-split wood, too. This activity is an extra-high calorie burner.

⌒ **Rake leaves.** In the fall, give your landscaper a vacation and rake your own leaves. Start a compost pile and you'll have a terrific soil amendment come spring.

⌒ **Take the stairs, not the elevator, if you can.**

.~ **Walk or bicycle to work.** If the distance is too far, park as far away as you safely can. Bicycling is a great way to commute, too.

.~ **Play with your children or grandchildren.** Don't just sit on the sidelines — get involved. The best exercises are those that bring the most enjoyment. Increased activity and fitness bring increased energy and stamina.

.~ **Learn to do two things at once.** If your treadmill or stationary bike has a magazine rack, read a magazine or book while you walk or pedal. Lift dumbbells while watching television.

.~ **Forgo unnecessary kitchen appliances.** Knead bread dough by hand instead of using a bread machine. Wash and dry dishes. Whip cream and beat cake batter with a whisk, not electric beaters. Chop vegetables with a knife, not the food processor.

.~ **Give yourself opportunities to walk.** Need to run two errands that happen to be in the same retail mall, but are located at opposite ends? Don't park and drive to each one, walk!

4
Care for Yourself, Naturally

If you keep active and nourish your body with healthful foods, it will reward you with gorgeous skin and hair. Pamper and cleanse your skin and hair with natural, gentle products to become your most radiant. By taking good care of yourself, inside and out, you'll not only feel fabulous but you'll look fabulous, too!

Unless you make all of your personal-care products yourself, you will have to do a bit of shopping to find pure, organic formulations. A few companies do make an effort to manufacture nearly natural products with minimal use of synthetic ingredients and preservatives. To find these and other natural products, visit your local health-food store and read lots of labels, or shop natural or herbal product catalogs. Be an educated consumer.

Let's Face It

Like it or not, the appearance and health of your facial skin, which includes the throat and décolletage, is what people notice first about you. Hairstyle takes second place. You can be wearing the most striking outfit but if your skin is gray, pimply, parched, red, irritated, flaky, or looking like an oil field, that beautiful ensemble will go unnoticed.

The number-one purpose of your skin is to act as a protective barrier. This tough yet tender barrier prevents the absorption of toxic chemicals shields against solar radiation, and protects against injury, while it also aids in sensory perception, regulates temperature, maintains moisture balance, manufactures vitamin D, assists in excreting wastes, and metabolizes and stores fat.

Essential Oil Blends for Healthy Skin

Quality pharmaceutical- and aromatherapeutic-grade essential oils are blessings from nature that help to nourish, balance, tone, and support all of the skin's functions. The specialty essential oils I prefer are unlike most essential oils available in today's health-food stores; they are distilled at much lower temperatures and many of the plants are · organically grown. (See Resources for mail-order catalogs that specialize in these essential oils.) If you want a superior skin-care product you must use superior ingredients.

The following formulas are extremely safe, can be used by people of almost all ages — except children under 2 years — and have no other contraindications.

Antiaging Treatment

This oil is recommended for mature, devitalized, environmentally damaged, or smoker's skin. All essential oils are specific for dry, chapped, sagging skin, and they will aid in cell regeneration.

> 2 teaspoons hazelnut oil
> 2 teaspoons unrefined (if available) rosehip seed oil
> 2 teaspoons unrefined avocado oil
> 2 drops balsam Peru *(Myroxylon balsamum* var. *pereirae)* essential oil
> 4 drops neroli *(Citrus aurantium)* essential oil
> 2 drops palmarosa *(Cymbopogon martini)* essential oil

2 drops rose otto *(Rosa damascena)* essential oil

1. Combine all ingredients in a 1-ounce, dark glass bottle and cap tightly with a screw-type top. Shake vigorously to blend. Store in a dark, cool, dry cabinet for 2 weeks prior to use so oils can synergize. It is important to not store a dropper top in the bottle, as the rubber will degrade and allow the volatile therapeutic properties of the essential oils to evaporate. Reserve a separate dropper top just for this bottle. For maximum potency, use within 6 months.

2. To use, first cleanse the skin with a mild, super-fatted goat milk or herbal soap or a natural creamy cleanser of your choice. Then place 3 to 5 drops of oil in your palm, mix with a dab of facial cream if desired, and massage into face and throat for 1 minute. Do this twice daily.

Yield: Approximately 1 ounce

Calming and Restorative Skin Treatment

This treatment is recommended for healthy oily skin; irritated, sensitive, inflamed, or acneic skin; and skin suffering from rosacea, eczema, or psoriasis.

> 2 teaspoons kukui nut or hazelnut oil
>
> 4 teaspoons commercial organic aloe vera juice
>
> 2 drops Moroccan blue chamomile *(Tanacetum annuum)* essential oil
>
> 2 drops ylang ylang *(Cananga odorata)* essential oil
>
> 2 drops patchouli *(Pogostemon cablin)* essential oil
>
> 2 drops cedarwood *(Juniperus virginiana)* essential oil
>
> 2 drops myrtle *(Myrtus communis)* essential oil

See Antiaging Treatment recipe (page 114) for directions for usage and storage.

Yield: Approximately 1 ounce

Time Waits for No Woman

Realize this: 90 percent of all visible signs of aging are preventable. The other 10 percent is genetic. It's easy to blame your parents for your big nose, but you can't always blame them for your wrinkles. With proper care of the skin and your overall health you can look much younger than your years. The clock may say you're 50 years old, but physically you may look and feel 40.

For Skin That's Beautifully Smooth, Clean, and Clear

The following is a list of my tried-and-true favorite skin-care items and ingredients.

~ **Oats and cream.** This is my favorite facial cleanser; I recommend it for all skin types. Simply grind a handful of old-fashioned oats in a nut/seed grinder until you have the consistency of coarsely ground oat flour. Measure out a tablespoon or two into a small bowl and add enough heavy cream to form a paste. (If your skin is oily, use water or skim milk instead of heavy cream.) Allow mixture to thicken for a minute. Using your fingers, massage the cleanser onto the face, throat, and chest in circular motions for a minute. Rinse with cool water. Follow with moisturizer, if necessary. *Beauty note:* Straight heavy cream is a terrific eye makeup remover.

⌒ **Super-fatted goat's milk soap.** If you have an oily or seasonally oily complexion, this type of soap is perfect for removing excess oil without stripping your skin dry. I use a bar of herbal scented soap — available in some health-food stores and through September's Sun Herbal Soap & Skin Care Company (see Resources) — during the hot and humid summer months.

⌒ **Topical vitamin C.** Vitamin C creams and gels are touted as being able to smooth fine lines and wrinkles by penetrating the skin and protecting against free-radical formation. But the main reason I like these products is that they maximize the effectiveness of sunscreen if worn as a first layer of protection.

Warning: Many of the topical vitamin C skin-care products on the market today are worthless. Vitamin C is highly unstable and loses its potency rapidly. What you want to look for on the label is this: a 5 to 15 percent concentration of L-ascorbic acid (a stable form of vitamin C) in an acidic or low-pH formula base. Antioxidants and lipids should also be listed as ingredients; these are additional stabilizers and they delay aging of the skin. The container should be an airtight dispenser, which prevents product breakdown.

~ **Raw apple cider vinegar.** This vinegar contains malic acid, a naturally occurring alpha-hydroxy acid that helps slough off dead skin cells. After cleansing, pat the face dry. Then saturate a cotton pad with a solution of 1 part vinegar to 1 part water and apply to face, throat, and chest, as you would a toner. It may be used full-strength if you have oily skin, but it should be diluted for normal or normal-to-oily skin types. Avoid if you have dry or sensitive skin.

~ **Unripe papaya.** This beautiful tropical fruit is full of natural beta-hydroxy acid and the "meat tenderizing" enzyme papain. The mashed pulp, applied in a thin layer over a clean face, throat, and chest, as a wet mask, will help even out skin tone and soften skin. Lie down and rest for 10 to 20 minutes, then rinse with cool water. Pat dry, and follow with moisturizer if necessary. It may be used once a week. Papaya is especially useful for a fading tan or dry, flaky, rough skin. If it gets into your eyes, rinse with copious amounts of water to avoid stinging. If you can't find unripe papaya, ripe is fine.

~ **Yogurt.** Full of lactic acid, an alpha-hydroxy acid, yogurt is fabulous for a quick and gentle skin smoothie — especially for highly sensitive skin. It removes surface dead-skin cells, leaving skin refreshed and exfoliated. Simply apply a thin layer of plain, organic yogurt to your clean face, throat, and chest. Lie down and rest for 10 to 20 minutes. Rinse with cool water. Pat dry, and follow with moisturizer if necessary. Use every day if desired. Yogurt will often normalize an uneven skin tone and slightly fade freckles over time.

~ **Alpha-hydroxy acids.** These acids occur naturally in foods. They dissolve the bond that holds dead skin cells together and increase hydration, resulting in super-smooth skin that actually looks younger and exhibits fewer fine lines.

Found in lotions and creams formulated for face or body care (available from better drug stores or department stores), the acid(s) in these products gently slough off rough skin without the use of an abrasive. Start with a 5 percent solution, applied once a day after cleansing. Slowly, over a period of several weeks, advance to an 8 to 10 percent solution if necessary. If no irritation develops, use until you see smoother, more evenly textured skin. Prolonged use will tend to fade age spots, but it will not remove them. *Note:* Wear a strong sunscreen after application, as alpha-hydroxy acids thin the skin and increase sun sensitivity.

~ **Clay mask.** The clay mask is an ancient method of tightening the skin, stimulating circulation, removing impurities, and depositing minerals into the tissues. French green clay and cosmetic white clay are available from most health food stores. Mix a tablespoon of clay with enough water to make a spreadable paste. Apply it to your clean face, throat, and chest, and allow to dry. Rinse with cool water. Follow with a moisturizer. Use once a week.

~ **Organic oils.** No matter what your skin type, maintaining proper hydration levels as you age is vital to your skin's health. I use unrefined, expeller-pressed, organically produced vegetable, nut, and seed oils to seal in precious moisture. Before bed, apply a thin coating of organic oil to your clean, damp face, neck, and chest and massage in circular motions until absorbed (see page 122).

Skin Health, Stress Management, or Sheer Indulgence?

Try to have a facial every month. This will calm your nerves, drain away muscle tension, and also assist in maintaining perfectly clean pores and appropriate skin moisture balance and tone. A knowledgeable esthetician will be able to guide you to various salon or at-home treatments that can help erase or fade those minor skin imperfections that may be bothering you.

Beneficial Organic Oils

Oil	Recommended Use
Jojoba	All skin types
Sesame	Normal and dry skin
Neem	Severely dry skin, eczema, and psoriasis
Hazelnut	All skin types
Sea buckthorn*	Mature, dry, or environmentally damaged skin

*One of the richest sources of antioxidant vitamins E and A, this bright orange, nourishing oil is high in essential fatty acids, particularly rare palmitoleic acid (a constituent of the skin's sebum). Aubrey Organics (see Resources), manufacturers a line of products utilizing this fabulous oil. I highly recommend trying these formulations.

Be Sun Savvy

Admit it. On a gorgeous spring or summer day, the warmth of the sun feels good on your skin. It simply makes you feel good all over. The sun is not the enemy the media would have you believe. It is necessary for all life on this planet, including yours. It also facilitates the development of vitamin D within the skin, helping your body to more effectively absorb calcium. I believe that 10 to 15 minutes a day of unprotected sun exposure before 10:30 A.M. or after 4:30 P.M. is essential for mental and physical health.

The problem is not the sun itself but excessive exposure to the sun's rays. Repeated, unprotected daily exposure to the sun for 20 minutes or more can do as much harm to your skin as a blistering sunburn. The occurrence of skin cancer is rising dramatically, despite media and medical cautions to wear sunscreen daily. There are several reasons for the increase, from improper use of sunscreen products (always follow label instructions and purchase a new sunscreen every year) to products that offer protection only from UVB rays (UVA rays are up to 1,000 times more intense).

Don't Rely on SPF

Did you know that the SPF (sun protection factor) rating you see on a sunscreen label indicates only the level of UVB protection, not UVA protection? Further, the SPF rating does not acknowledge the specific amount of absorption of the UVB rays, so it doesn't really tell you how well your sunscreen will perform.

SPF ratings may also give a false sense of security. For instance, if your unprotected skin burns in 30 minutes and you choose to wear a sunscreen with a SPF of 15, the label suggests that you can stay outside 15 times your burning time limit, or 7.5 hours, before you begin to burn. While it may be true that you won't visibly burn in that amount of time, you cannot stay out in the sun all day and not receive some type of skin damage. Remember that the sun's effects are cumulative. Always use caution. Sunscreens will help reduce the risk of additional damage to your skin, and they may help turn the tide on premature aging, sagging, and wrinkling of the skin; however, they *cannot* repair damage caused by years of unprotected exposure to the sun.

To date in the United States, there is no definitive measure that manufacturers can use to inform consumers about how much UVB and UVA absorption is truly being offered in the particular product. The FDA is currently working to improve the information presented on sunscreen labels.

Lip Service

Often dry, with thin skin and no oil glands for lubrication — that pretty much defines your lips. Depending upon the degree of environmental and synthetic lipstick-ingredient exposure or prescription drug side effects, lips frequently suffer unnecessary stress. My favorite, cost-efficient natural lip conditioner is cocoa butter. Available for under $2 from your local drug store, a small tube of lip-loving, pure cocoa butter will give your lips a slight cocoa-flavored sheen. Wear plain or as a conditioning base for that favorite $15 tube of fabulously frosted, yet highly drying, red designer lipstick.

Your Body Beautiful

Many of the skin-care recommendations I've made also apply to the care of your body. Admittedly, facial treatments are designed to be gentler, but if the skin covering your entire body is delicate and sensitive you may be better off using facial-care products from head to toe.

This section focuses primarily on the simple and natural care of body skin, preserving the protective barrier while gently cleansing, sloughing, and moisturizing the outer layer. Fabulous-looking skin feels fabulous, too.

Smooth-as-Silk Herbal Body Oils

As you age, your skin becomes drier for three reasons. First, your skin naturally becomes thinner from losing its protective fat layer, thus it can't hold in as much water and softening lipids (fats). Second, lubricating sebum, your skin's natural protective oil, is no longer produced at the same rate as when you were in your teens and twenties. Third, your skin has been exposed to decades of environmental damage, such as excess sun, artificial heat and cold, and pollution — all of which have altered the skin's structure, leaving it more sensitive.

I've developed two bath and body oil dry-skin remedies that work like a charm to combat even the flakiest of skin. Here's the rub: In order for these formulas to work properly, you'll need to drink at least 8 glasses of purified water daily, avoid smoking, minimize caffeine and alcohol consumption, and use a loofah or natural-bristled body brush daily to slough off dry-skin buildup prior to bathing. See page 131 for more information on dry-skin brushing.

Mineral-Rich Herbs

Herbs that are excellent for overall nourishment of skin, hair, and nails include:

⟿ Alfalfa	⟿ Nettle
⟿ Borage	⟿ Oat straw
⟿ Burdock root	⟿ Red clover
⟿ Chamomile	⟿ Red raspberry
⟿ Horsetail	⟿ Thyme

Anti-inflammatory Treatment Oil

This formula is specifically designed for those of you suffering from eczema and psoriasis, or sunburned, wind burned, rashy, dry, flaky, cracked, or irritated skin. All oils should be organic, cold-pressed, and unrefined, if possible.

> ½ cup hazelnut oil
> 2 tablespoons jojoba oil
> 1 tablespoon flaxseed oil
> 1 tablespoon avocado oil
> ¼ cup extra-virgin, first-pressing olive oil
> 10 drops Moroccan blue chamomile *(Tanacetum annuum)* essential oil
> 10 drops calendula extract (CO_2) *(Calendula officinalis)*
> 10 drops helichrysum *(Helichrysum italicum* var. serotinum) essential oil
> 10 drops eucalyptus *(Eucalyptus citriodora)* essential oil

Combine all ingredients in an 8-ounce, dark glass bottle. Store in a cool, dry, dark cabinet for 2 weeks before use. Shake well before each application. For maximum freshness, use formula within 6 months.

To use as a body oil: Apply approximately 1 tablespoon (more or less according to body size) after toweling off from a bath or shower. Massage the oil into your feet and work your way up to your neck. Towel off any excess, then wait 10 minutes before dressing.

To use as a bath oil: First soak for 5 minutes, then add 2 teaspoons of oil to bath water. Swish water with hands to blend. Soak for about 20 minutes more. Towel dry and apply additional moisturizer, if necessary.

Store oil in refrigerator for up to a year. May be stored at room temperature if used within two months.

Yield: 8 ounces

Bonus: This formula is excellent for the treatment of bruised skin. The first three essential oils (that is, Moroccan blue chamomile, calendula extract, and helichrysum) are superior anti-inflammatories and help heal bruises quickly if a few drops of formula are applied immediately following injury. Reapply several times per day until the bruise disappears.

Velvet Skin Oil

This is a basic skin-nourishing oil blend that's good for all skin types. The hemp seed oil is high in essential fatty acids, while the sesame oil is a natural antioxidant and low-SPF sunscreen.

½ cup food-grade hemp seed oil

½ cup sesame oil (not the toasted variety)

10 drops geranium *(Pelargonium graveolens)* essential oil

10 drops Roman chamomile *(Anthemis nobilis)* essential oil

10 drops lavender *(Lavandula angustifolia)* essential oil

See Anti-Inflammatory Treatment Oil (page 128) for instructions.

Yield: 8 ounces

Get Rid of the Rough Stuff

Wouldn't it be nice to just peel off all our old skin to expose a new, baby-soft layer that's free of blemishes, dry patches, and age spots? Dead skin cells fall away from your body on a daily basis, but every 28 to 45 days, depending on age, your body builds an entirely new layer of skin. The older you get, the slower the turnover of new skin cells.

Dry, flaky, dull skin is a sure sign of old age. Remember, youthful skin is moist, glowing, and silky. You can attain younger looking skin by performing exfoliating procedures at least twice per week. By getting rid of this outer layer of dead skin-cell buildup, your moisturizer will actually be able to penetrate, thereby doing a better job at keeping your skin soft and moisture-laden. The following techniques will definitely improve the health of your skin. Try them!

~ **Sisal cloth.** This is a rough, abrasive cloth woven from a fibrous plant material that is terrific for exfoliating the arms and legs.

~ **Skin brushing.** The skin is your body's largest — and often neglected — organ of elimination, ridding the body daily of up to two pounds of waste materials, such as dead skin, urea, salts, minerals, sebum, and perspiration. If the skin is not able to carry out its normal detoxification function, the other elimination organs suffer additional burdens. Conversely, if you can improve the function of the skin, you will improve the functioning of the other elimination organs.

Before bathing, brush dry skin, using circular motions, with a dry vegetable-fiber bath brush. Start at the soles of the feet and work up the legs and trunk to the heart. Then move from the palms of the hands up the arms and across the back and abdomen. Avoid the breasts and face. This procedure should take only 5 minutes. "When practiced daily for several months," Robert Gray, author of *The Colon Health Handbook* states, "skin brushing is very effective for improving body tone. Five minutes per day of skin brushing is easily worth thirty minutes of vigorous physical exercise in this respect."

~ **Salt and oil.** This simple exfoliating mixture is super-effective and quick to make. In a small bowl, combine a tablespoon of vegetable oil with a tablespoon sea salt, table salt, or granulated sugar. Shower for a few minutes in order to thoroughly moisten your skin. Massage the blend all over your body or simply where you feel you need a bit of exfoliation. Rinse well, pat dry, and end by applying your favorite moisturizer, if necessary. The oil in the mixture should leave your skin feeling soft and smooth.

~ **Alpha hydroxy acids.** See page 120 for description.

~ **Oats and sunflower seeds.** Do you have dry skin that's ultra sensitive? Make a gentle body scrub by grinding a quarter-cup old-fashioned oats and a quarter-cup raw sunflower seeds until a fine, granular consistency forms. In a small bowl, combine the dry ingredients with enough half and half or heavy cream until you have a spreadable paste. Prior to showering, stand in the shower stall and massage the mixture over your entire body. Use circular motions, and concentrate on massaging the driest parts. Do this for about 5 minutes. The scrub is gentle enough to be used on your face, if you wish. Rinse well with warm water and bathe as usual, or simply follow with your favorite moisturizer. This procedure can be done as often as desired. Leaves skin sleek, supple, and ultra soft.

Fabulous Hair Every Day

Bad hair days tend to put a real damper on your mood and self-esteem. This may sound incredibly superficial, but it's true: Beautiful, shiny, healthy, bouncy hair can boost your confidence and improve your image.

The right cut, suited to your lifestyle, facial shape, and natural hair texture is the first place to start. The wrong style, even though your hair may be healthy, won't bring out your good looks, so I suggest a few interviews with top stylists for suggestions before you decide.

Next, you need to determine the condition of your hair. Oily hair looks greasy within 24 hours after washing and is frequently limp with possible dandruff. Normal hair is not too oily or too dry and behaves as it should. Dry hair can suffer from an oily or dry scalp but have dry, brittle ends. This type has a tendency to be flyaway and doesn't shine as much as other hair types. Hair damaged by the sun, sea, pool, extreme temperatures, chemical processing, styling-aid use, or by medicines is dry, brittle, dull, unmanageable, and generally looks unhealthy.

Aging begins to take its toll on hair at about age 35. To what degree depends upon genetics and the various treatments or neglect to which you've subjected your hair over the years.

Add Life to Your Tresses

Natural hair treatments, in combination with a healthy diet and exercise, can help rejuvenate lifeless locks and normalize scalp conditions ranging from dandruff to overproduction of oil.

~ **Stimulate your scalp.** One of the main causes of dry hair is lack of circulation within the scalp. This prevents sebum and necessary nutrients from reaching the hair. Hair follicles can become clogged from dead skin buildup, hair spray, silicone in various styling aids, sebum buildup from lack of hygiene, and even stress. By doing 5 minutes of head and scalp massage every day, you'll soon see a shinier, softer, healthier head of hair.

~ **Help for the dried and fried.** To help quench your hair's thirst, try this fruity hair mask. It's great for all hair types except oily, and it makes enough for medium-length hair.

In a medium glass bowl, mash half of a ripe avocado with half of a ripe banana. Add 1 tablespoon of jojoba, avocado, flaxseed, or extra-virgin olive oil, and 3 drops lemon *(Citrus limon)* essential oil. Apply with hands to dry hair. Cover hair with a shower

3-Step Scalp Massage

1. Use a tablespoon of jojoba oil, a teaspoon at a time, as a massage oil. Or, simply place 2 drops of lavender *(Lavandula angustifolia)* essential oil and 2 drops of basil leaf *(Ocimum basilicum)* essential oil and a tablespoon of aloe vera juice in a small bowl. Stir briskly to blend, then use a teaspoon at a time to massage scalp. The latter blend does not have to be washed out and will not leave a greasy residue, while the jojoba oil is recommended for dry and/or damaged hair. You may also perform the massage with dry hands.

2. Bend over at the waist while standing or sitting. This increases circulation. Beginning at

cap or plastic bag and leave on for up to 60 minutes. Shampoo out, and follow with your favorite natural detangler, if necessary. Your hair should be soft, frizz-free, and shiny. For severely damaged hair, do this treatment up to 3 times per week.

the base of your neck, place fingertips beneath your hair and massage scalp using small, circular motions. Slowly move up and forward toward your forehead. Once you reach the forehead, reverse and return to the base of your neck.

3. Now, begin as you did above, but move up and over each ear toward your temples. When you reach the temples, do 10 very slow circular motions. You should feel the tension drain from your head. Reverse, and return to the base of your neck. This massage is also super for relief of tension headaches and insomnia.

Clean and Fresh Herbal Wash

Looking for a chemical-free alternative to the standard mass-produced shampoos and body washes? Do you have allergies or sensitivities that make choosing personal-care products difficult? Then this herb-scented, low-sudsing, multipurpose liquid is for you. It's a great shampoo and body wash and can be used as a hand soap, facial cleanser, or handy travel detergent.

1 tablespoon dried basil leaves

1 teaspoon chopped, dried marsh mallow root

1 tablespoon dried chamomile flowers

1 tablespoon dried lavender flowers

1 tablespoon dried sage leaves

½ teaspoon lecithin granules

4 cups boiling distilled water

4 ounces plain or scented liquid castile soap

¼ teaspoon jojoba oil

10 drops lavender *(Lavandula angustifolia)* essential oil

10 drops rosemary *(Rosmarinus officinalis,* chemotype *verbenon)* essential oil

10 drops peppermint *(Mentha piperita)* essential oil

10 drops basil leaf *(Ocimum basilicum)*
   essential oil

10 drops lemon *(Citrus limon)*
   essential oil

1. Boil water in a pot. Remove boiling water from heat; add herbs and lecithin. Stir to immerse ingredients. Cover and steep for 30 minutes.

2. Strain liquid into a medium-sized bowl. Really squeeze or press the herbs in order to extract every drop.

3. While gently stirring, slowly pour in the castile soap.

4. Add half of the jojoba and essential oils directly to each of two 16-ounce plastic squeeze bottles. Then pour in the soap mixture. Shake vigorously to blend. Store one bottle in the refrigerator until needed. The mixture will keep for up to 4 months if refrigerated or 1 month if left at room temperature.

5. To use, pour approximately 1 tablespoon of herbal shampoo into your palm. Massage the scalp well, then rinse thoroughly. Use as much as desired for a body wash.

Yield: Approximately 32 ounces

Eye-Opening Good Looks

Ever look in the mirror and think your "windows to the soul" resemble those of a college student's after pulling an "all nighter" before final exams? Eyes are expressive, our silent communicators of happiness, sadness, anger, fear, disappointment, longing, and love. Yet the eyes are ever so sensitive to environmental stresses, diet, and lifestyle factors. The eye area is one of the first to register your true age, since the skin directly beneath the eyes contains no sebaceous glands to lubricate it and it is extremely thin.

Send Eye Bags Packing and Erase Dark Circles

The *orbicularis oculi* is the muscle that opens and closes the eyelid. Improper application and removal of eye makeup, rubbing your eyes when irritated, insertion of contact lenses, squinting, or squishing your face into your bed pillow can all cause unnecessary stretching of this delicate muscle and its paper-thin skin covering. The result is a loss of elasticity, otherwise known as undereye bags, and dark circles. If you are genetically predisposed to having undereye bags and dark circles, these habits will only exacerbate the problem.

No time to pamper those peepers? Reach for camouflage makeup! In a pinch a creamy cover-up stick or pot of cream concealer will temporarily blend dark lines and circles and hide a blemish or two. A daily application of a sunscreen that is specifically designed for the face will help prevent the production of melanocytes (skin pigment cells) in the undereye area, which can enhance the already dark pigmentation.

If you wear eye makeup, you must use a super-effective, ultra-gentle eye makeup remover. I find that a good creamy facial cleanser, applied thickly with my ring finger over the entire eye area, works great. (A quality vegetable oil works if no cream cleanser is available.) Allow the cleanser to remain on the eye area for about a minute to dissolve the makeup, then gently swipe the makeup from your eyes using a damp cotton pad. Begin at the inner corner of your eye, wipe up and over your eyelid out to the outer corner, then inward beneath the lower row of lashes back toward the inner corner. This method causes the least amount of pulling on the eye skin and musculature.

I highly recommend the use of a good herbal eye cream or gel to fight dryness and provide a "lifted" appearance. For maximum benefit, this product should be worn morning and night. Look for ingredients —

Say Goodbye to Eye Fatigue

Sleep is the world's best beauty secret. Nothing — absolutely nothing — will put the sparkle back into your stressed-out eyes like a good night's rest! Enough said?

A few years ago I was introduced to a method of stress reduction called "cupping." It is a simple yet amazingly effective way to relieve eyestrain and mild headaches, as well as relax facial muscles and calm the mind. Sit while performing this therapy. Prepare for relaxation by taking three deep breaths through your nose, expanding your lower

such as vitamin C, aloe vera gel, jojoba oil, apricot kernel oil, sorbitol, squalene, hydrolyzed mucopolysaccharides, extracts of chamomile, eyebright, marshmallow, cucumber, ivy, calendula, arnica, licorice, fennel, or sambucus — listed on the label with minimal preservatives.

abdomen, and holding for 5 counts. Exhale slowly. Now rub the palms of your hands together rapidly until they are quite warm. Close your eyes and cup your warmed palms over your eyes, allowing them to receive the relaxing heat and rest out of the light. Be sure you're not pressing your hands into your eyes; just cup over them, leaving air space between your hands and eyes. Stay in this position for 1 or 2 minutes, then slowly open your fingers. Let your eyes feel the light on the eyelids. Remove your hands and open your eyes.

Reduce the Puffiness

Puffy eyes, sorry to say, are usually hereditary, but you can exert an amazing amount of control over this unsightly condition. Here's how.

~ **Increase your daily water consumption to a *minimum* of 6 to 8 glasses per day.** A dehydrated body actually retains water, and it shows up on your face and body as a swollen appearance.

~ **Use a gel-filled ice mask.** A gel-filled ice mask, kept in the freezer until needed, is an effective weapon against puffiness. Many women swear by these little masks as a surefire complexion and energy pick-me-up. They're also nice if you have a headache.

~ **Chill your facial moisturizer and eye cream, especially in the summer months.** This makes for an eye-soothing, refreshing application. Soaked and chilled green tea bags and black tea bags actually work wonders; the natural tannins help temporarily tighten slack skin, giving your eye area a youthful lift.

~ **Avoid salty foods.** They lead to water retention in your skin tissues.

~ **Minimize or eliminate alcohol intake.** Alcohol consumption can cause abnormal swelling of the eye tissue and discoloration under the eye as a result of expanding and contracting capillaries.

~ **Hide inside during peak allergy season.** Airborne allergens, such as dust, mold, and pollen, are common eye irritants. During peak allergy season, stay indoors if possible or at least exercise indoors. Avoid yard and garden work when the allergen counts are high. Rinsing the eyes with cool water several times per day can bring immediate relief, as can some brands of over-the-counter eye drops. Consult your pharmacist for the best brand for frequent use.

The Matter at Hand

Think about it: Over a lifetime, your hands are probably used more than all other body parts combined, with the possible exception of the heart and eyes. You literally "talk" with your hands to express emotion. Your hands work hard for you in the garden, doing yard work, mountain climbing, playing an instrument, lifting weights, typing, and writing. They give and receive vital sensory information all day, every day.

Because we use them constantly, our hands take lots of abuse. If you subjected your delicate facial skin to daily washings with harsh dish detergent, antibacterial soap, acidic and caustic household cleansers, garden grime, infant and animal messes, boiling water, hot kitchen utensils, and grease splatters, it would resemble a wrinkled prune in no time flat!

A Handful of Healing Hints

A woman's hands will frequently look older than her years unless she lavishes them with TLC. Let me pass along a few of my tried-and-true hand-health tips.

~ **Manicure.** Performed by a licensed nail technician, a manicure is recommended twice a year not only for a hand pampering and stress reduction session, but also for a professional checkup of nail, cuticle, and skin condition. A skilled nail tech can make even the most weathered, time-ravaged hands and nails look terrific again.

~ **Sunscreen.** According to Norma Pasekoff Weinberg, author of *Natural Hand Care*, "Photoaging of the skin (rough, leathery texture, sagging skin, and brown-pigmented, freckle-like spots on the back of the hands) is caused by undue exposure to sunlight. Long-term sun exposure degrades the skin's support network of collagen and elastin fibers and causes the skin to become less flexible." I recommend that you slather your hands with a thick layer of moisturizing sunscreen every time you wash your hands. It should be used in place of your regular hand cream, and a container should be placed by every sink in the house.

~ **Diamond dust nail file.** Toss those old-fashioned emery boards in the trash and invest in this type of nail maintenance tool to gently file away rough and peeling edges and snags. A cheap file can actually rip and tear your nails, leading to breakage.

 ⌒ **Gloves.** Wear gloves when gardening or doing outdoor chores to protect your hands from wear and tear and block the sun's rays.

 ⌒ **Slough.** It's important to remove dull, dead skin at least once a week if you want your moisturizer to do its job. In a small bowl, simply mix a tablespoon of sugar or salt with an equal amount of vegetable oil. Stir to coat grains. Gently massage hands, fingers, and web spaces thoroughly, rinse, and pat dry.

 ⌒ **Lighten those sun spots.** While sunscreen can help prevent future age spot formation, a 10 percent alpha-hydroxy acid hand lotion can aid in the erasure or lightening of unwanted pigmentation and rough texture. Ask your esthetician or nail technician for product recommendations.

 ⌒ **Condition.** To soften and condition the skin of your hands and maintain healthy cuticles, a nightly massage using 1 teaspoon of warm jojoba, almond, or castor oil combined with 1 drop of rosemary, lemon, or peppermint essential oil will do the trick.

Massage oil into damp hands for maximum absorption, then sleep in cotton gloves. You'll awaken with revitalized hands.

〜 **Buff, buff, buff.** Once a week, apply a drop of castor oil to each nail, massage in, and then, using a professional hand-held nail buffer, polish your nails to a healthy sheen. Gentle buffing stimulates circulation within the nail bed and can speed nail growth.

Be Sweet to Your Feet

"Wet foot, Dry foot, High foot, Low foot," says my young nephew Joshua as he reads his favorite book, *The Foot Book* by Dr. Seuss. You know, it's never too early to start taking good care of your feet.

Feet are amazingly tough, yet still particularly tender. A masterpiece of design, the foot contains some 33 joints, 112 ligaments, 26 bones (both feet contain a quarter of the bones in your entire body), and a complicated network of blood vessels, muscles, tendons, and nerves. All of these interrelated parts enable you to move with the balance and grace of a ballerina or with the speed and agility of an Olympic high-jumper.

Osteoarthritis

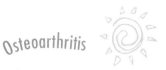

A degenerative form of arthritis, osteoarthritis affects twice as many women as men and can show up in the feet first. It is the result of years of joint stress, injury, and everyday wear and tear. It causes a degeneration of the cartilage in the joints and minor inflammation. The small joints in your feet are particularly vulnerable, due to the load they must carry daily. Symptoms of osteoarthritis can include stiffness and pain in the joints after heavy exercise, during damp or cold weather, or after you arise in the morning. It usually affects one or more joints.

As you get older, years of neglect, the wearing of improperly designed or poor-quality shoes, everyday living and exercise, medications, and illness can take their toll on your "dogs," leaving them barking for attention.

What can be done to prevent osteoarthritis from occurring or at least slow its progression? Always purchase proper-fitting footwear. Maintain normal weight; excess pounds add stress to weight-bearing joints, setting the stage for potential foot problems. Stay active and limber. Keep your feet dry and warm. And if your joints do feel stiff and sore, take a nice, warm foot bath, dry your feet thoroughly, apply a deep-heating mentholated cream, put on socks, and take a load off for awhile!

If symptoms continue to worsen, make an appointment with a podiatrist or health-care practitioner as soon as possible.

A Step in the Right Direction

If your feet don't feel good and function as they should, neither will you. A daily task as simple as walking can become a chore. Don't take your feet for granted. If you want to be comfortable and active late in life, then your feet need lifelong care.

~ **Keep calluses and other rough spots under control with regular maintenance.** Use a pumice stone, pediwand, or abrasive foot scrub as needed. If allowed to remain unchecked, hard, thickened areas can become painful, dry, cracked, or infected, making walking difficult. Engage the services of a licensed nail technician if you are unable to attend to necessary maintenance. See a podiatrist or chiropodist for concerns outside the nail tech's expertise, such as bunions, severely thickened calluses, hammertoes, corns, fungus, infection, and diabetic problems.

~ **Relax and relieve even the most tested feet by taking a nice, warm foot bath.** Add a cup of marbles to the water and roll your feet around atop the marbles to stimulate nerve endings. Pick up marbles with your toes, flex and contract feet and toes, and then release the marbles to stretch arches and muscles. If the weather outside is hot, use cool water in your foot bath.

~ **Solicit the help of a friend or significant other to give you a foot massage.** As far as I'm concerned, a hard, vigorous lower-leg and foot massage just can't be beat. It sends me into deep relaxation mode almost immediately. Purchase a bottle of peppermint foot lotion or add 2 to 4 drops of peppermint essential oil to a tablespoon of your favorite lotion for a scentsational moisturizing treat for your feet.

— **Moisturize.** The skin on the soles of your feet, like your palms, contains no sebaceous (oil) glands to lubricate and soften, leaving moisturizing up to you. Slather on a thick coat of cream each night before bed or before working out, put on natural-fiber socks, and let the conditioning ingredients pamper your piggies.

— **Measure your feet.** Don't assume you will wear the same size shoe from year to year. The shape of your feet changes with age, reflecting the cumulative affects of pregnancy and various types of daily impact. In fact, by age 45 your feet may be a whole size larger than they were in your early 20s. Feet tend to widen and lengthen with age. Make sure you have your feet measured while standing — not sitting — every time you buy shoes.

— **Get new shoes.** Worn-out shoes have lost their support mechanisms, which can lead to foot, leg, and back fatigue and problems. If you exercise frequently or your job demands that you be on your feet all day, it is paramount that you replace your shoes at least every 6 months.

Relax and Revitalize with Reflexology

This natural healing technique is based on the idea that there are reflexes in your feet and hands that correspond to your internal organs and body functions. Applying firm but gentle pressure with your thumbs and forefingers to certain points can relieve stress, improve circulation, and relax your mind.

A weekly session performed by a certified reflexologist is well worth the investment. Utilizing acupressure-like techniques combined with loosening movements, gentle twisting, and massage, reflexology will activate the healing powers of the body and promote a profound sense of well-being and deep relaxation. I highly recommend it to everyone. Many books are available on this subject so that you may learn to practice reflexology on yourself or your friends and family.

Finger Circling Relaxation Treatment

This massage technique is generally performed by the practitioner prior to and immediately after an entire reflexology session to promote relaxation and energy flow. Practice it on your own feet by sitting in a chair and crossing the ankle of one leg over the knee of the other, then grasping the foot with both hands (placing the thumbs on the midsole region and the fingers on top of the foot). Treat both feet equally. Use cream, oil, or lotion on the feet if desired.

Begin by placing your fingers at the base of the toes. Using tiny circular movements, massage the entire top of the foot, making sure to work your fingertips down between the phalanges and metatarsal bones. Don't forget the sides of the foot and around the anklebone. Then work your way back up the foot to the base of the toes. This massage technique is terrific for people who suffer from poor circulation or edema in their feet, as it stimulates the lymphatic system.

5

Awaken Your Spirit

My husband, Bill, and I recently visited the gardens of one of our customers, the Pilkingtons. As Bill discussed business with Mr. Pilkington, Mrs. Pilkington and I wandered through her gardens discussing plants, the pros and cons of natural plant mutations, plant cutting propagation, and my longing for a greenhouse. That morning I found a true kindred spirit; I was deeply moved. As our meeting with this lovely couple came to a close, Bill had a good job to put on our business schedule, and I was the buoyant recipient of a red lobelia plant, a spike of mature seedpods, a three-foot Kousa dogwood sapling, and a new friend.

Our elders have much wisdom to offer. Nurture your spirit whenever you can, by reaching out to them and to your family, friends, and neighbors.

Reconnect with Your Community

As we hurdle through our increasingly busy and high-tech lives — benefactors of faster forms of communication, with immediate access to staggering amounts of information and automated everything — a new problem is rearing its ugly head: technological isolation. Are we gradually losing the warmth of human touch and voice; the fulfillment of physical, emotional, and spiritual intimacy; the feeling of belonging to a community? In a word, yes — unless we take steps to embrace the advances in technology while remembering to integrate our instinctive need for real human involvement in our lives.

People Need People

Feeling disconnected with modern society, with your community, even with your neighbors? You're not alone. The frustration with mechanization, depersonalization, alienation, and loss of the friendly human voice and touch is steadily mounting. Throughout history, people have been involved in relationships with other people.

It's a fact of life: Humans are social creatures and, as such, we have an innate need to be involved with other people in all aspects of life.

Psychologist Abraham Maslow developed his now-famous Hierarchy of Needs in the late 1960s. Beyond the basic human needs for air, water, food, and sex, he described five broader layers. The second, third, and fourth of these needs are relevant to our discussion.

~ **Physiological needs.** These include the basics I mentioned above, plus sodium, sugar, protein, vitamins and minerals, as well as the maintenance of the correct pH balance and a stable body temperature. We also need adequate rest, warmth, protection from the elements, activity, avoidance of pain, and bodily waste removal.

~ **Security and safety needs.** When the first layer of physiological needs are met, we also desire a safe neighborhood in which to live and work, or at least a safe home and circumstances surrounding our lives, including job stability and possibly retirement security.

Love, affection, and belonging needs. In the third layer, we feel the need for friendships, children, a spouse, general affection from relationships, a need for community, and a sense of belonging. There is a strong need to escape alienation and loneliness and to give love and affection.

 Esteem needs. In this layer, the person looks for self-esteem, and a high level of self-respect from others in order to feel valuable in the community, self-confident, competent, independent, and free.

 Self-actualization needs. This layer is an ongoing process. We become devoted to something very precious to us — a calling, perhaps. We need to do and be what we were born to be, whether an artist, a writer, poet, musician, engineer, or architect. If this need is not met, a feeling of edginess, restlessness, or tension will develop.

In addition to the emotional and spiritual blessings of person-to-person interaction, there are health benefits, too. People who have strong support networks have a higher survival rate from heart attacks, reduced rates of depression and anxiety, and are less susceptible to the common cold than those who have no one to turn to for support. The Mayo Foundation for Medical Education and Research suggests that maintaining social ties fosters better self-care, improves self-esteem, and gives meaning and purpose to your life. It's even theorized that social support may boost the immune system, contributing to better general health.

Expand Your Social Network

There are a number of ways to gain new friends and strengthen your existing friendships. Try some.

~ **Gather together.** At your church, your community center, a neighborhood park, or even your own home, schedule a regular potluck dinner or a simple gathering for members in your community or neighborhood to come visit, discuss issues, share information, play games, or just get to know each other.

~ **Join a group or club.** Get involved and stay busy with other like-minded people. There are many groups listed in the local newspaper, on store bulletin boards, or even on the Internet. Build social ties by joining walking, gardening, craft, book discussion, sports or political groups.

～ **Start a weekly or monthly lunch meeting with your friends to catch up on the latest happenings and concerns.** Remember, maintaining a friendship requires a commitment of time and psychological intimacy. Close friends are too valuable a commodity to let slip by the wayside.

～ **Teach a class.** Are you an expert at something? Many women like to teach adult education classes in fields ranging from computer technology to aromatherapy, from painting to furniture refinishing. You'll soon become a respected member of the community, sought after for your expertise in your field.

～ **Remember important dates.** Never forget birthdays, anniversaries, graduations, a new birth in the family, or get-well or sympathy cards. Organize your calendar in January and list all important dates for the year so you won't forget. It's important, and it shows you really care!

～ **Learn to confide in others and open yourself to others and they will frequently confide in you.** This soon forms a close-knit bond between you and your friends. Be sure to listen to others; make them feel that you sincerely care about how they're doing.

~ **Volunteer.** To truly awaken your spirit for benefit of yourself *and* others, volunteer to work for charity organizations, such as Toys For Tots, Salvation Army, Big Brothers Big Sisters of America, local soup kitchens and homeless shelters, local hospitals or nursing homes, or Meals on Wheels. Your kindness will be remembered.

~ **Commune with animals.** If you love dogs, organize an early-morning or evening dog-walking group. The dogs will be intrigued by the new scents of their neighborhood pals, you and your pet will get plenty of needed exercise, and you'll meet new friends with common interests.

~ **Take a class.** Interested in learning something new? Broaden your mind as well as your social base by taking a class.

~ **Be a greeter.** Welcome each new person or family in your neighborhood with an old-fashioned basket of goodies. Introduce yourself, and if received warmly let them know where you live and invite them to visit for tea or coffee sometime.

Connect with Your Family

If you live near family members, consider yourself lucky. It's much easier to stop and visit than if you live hundreds or thousands of miles away. Even still, with everyone's busy schedules these days, it can be difficult to arrange these get-togethers. My mother-in-law lives only 3 miles away but works 6 days a week, like I do, so we have to make a conscious effort to call each other as often as possible, send letters and e-mails, have dinner, celebrate the holidays together, and stop by for brief visits.

In centuries past, cultures such as the Japanese, Italian, Spanish, and Chinese traditionally relied on extended families or entire communities for help with child rearing, education, harvesting of food, and provision of shelter. The Native Americans, prior to the white man's invasion, lived in tribes or extended communities for the benefit of all involved. The American farming community of today, though it is rapidly dwindling, is usually a close-knit group of several generations who help run the family business, share in child- and elder-care responsibilities, and spend holidays together.

Like many of you, I have family members that live thousands of miles away, scattered throughout the country. I like to use e-mail as often as possible to leave a message of encouragement, congratulations, gratitude, or simply an "I'm thinking of you" note. For relatives who don't yet have access to this technology, a good, old-fashioned phone call does the trick. And, personally, I love letter writing. It's so intimate. Receiving a letter from someone means a lot to me. I know that they had to take precious time from their schedule to think about me and pen their thoughts. Just touching the writing makes me feel special.

Family reunions are a good way to get in touch with everyone at the same time. My father organized one a few years ago at a retreat center in the scenic Smokey Mountains of north Georgia over the Thanksgiving holiday. It was a blast! Many of the cousins that I hadn't seen in 20 years were there with their children. I loved catching up with everyone.

The key to togetherness, whether long-distance or local, with family or friends, is simply determining your priorities. Imagine

We'd love your thoughts . . .

Your reactions, criticisms, things you did or didn't like about this Storey Book. Please use space below (or write a letter if you'd prefer — even send photos!) telling how you've made use of the information . . . how you've put it to work . . . the more details the better!

Thanks in advance for your help in building our library of good Storey Books.

Pamela B. Art

Publisher, Storey Books

Book Title: _____

Purchased From: _____

Comments: _____

_____

_____

_____

_____

_____

Your Name: _____

Mailing Address: _____

E-mail Address: _____

☐ Please check here if you'd like our latest Storey's Books for Country Living Catalog, (or call 800-441-5700 to order).

☐ You have my permission to quote from my comments and use these quotations in ads, brochures, mail, and other promotions used to market Storey Books.

Signed _____ Date _____

e-mail=thoughts@storey.com   www.storeybooks.com   * Printed in the USA   07/00

From: _____

BUSINESS REPLY MAIL

FIRST-CLASS MAIL   PERMIT NO. 2   POWNAL VT

POSTAGE WILL BE PAID BY ADDRESSEE

STOREY'S BOOKS FOR COUNTRY LIVING
STOREY COMMUNICATIONS INC
RR1 BOX 105
POWNAL VT   05261-9988

if we put relationships first ahead of financial success, career advancement, and multiple accomplishments. What would your world be like?

Feed Your Soul

Are you a giver? Always nurturing, caring, and providing for everyone but you? That describes my dear mother to a T. She maintains a full schedule of volunteer work in hospitals, nursing homes, and church functions. But I occasionally hear her mention that she has very little time to devote to her passions, such as gardening, embroidery, sewing, and painting. It's important not to neglect yourself in your giving.

In my book *50 Simple Ways to Pamper Yourself*, I relate the benefits of taking time out just for *you*. If you want to live a long, joyous, well-rounded life, you must dedicate some time each day — or at least each week — to nurture *your* soul, *your* passions, *your* desires. Otherwise you'll be 90 years old before you know it and asking yourself, "Why didn't I do this or learn to do that? Where did all the years go?"

Nothing can replace what can be acted out in a personal sensory relationship.

—LINDA MARKS

You Deserve It!

For the sake of your health and sanity, learn to feed your soul the food it yearns for. And take time out to pamper yourself, as well.

If the head and body are to be well, you must begin by curing the soul.

—PLATO

∼ **Take a day off to do what you love!** Go antiquing, to a museum, or to flea markets, or go picnicking in a public garden. A change of scenery will do you good!

∼ **Clear your head, revitalize your body, and let go of the guilt.** Partake of sheer indulgences. Book a "day of well-being" at the local day spa. After a facial, pedicure, manicure, reflexology session, and herbal body wrap, your skin will glow and your mind will be wondering why you didn't do this a long time ago.

∼ **Once a month, visit a massage therapist or reiki practitioner for an hour of deep relaxation.** If you're a constant "giver", allow someone else to give her healing energy back to you. You'll be amazed at how rejuvenated you feel.

∼ **Give new meaning to the phrase "older and wiser."** Learn a new skill or two! Go to your local library and check out language tapes. Teach yourself to speak Italian or sign up for an adult education class in a discipline you've always wanted to study.

~ **Write a letter.** Seems letter writing is going the way of the dinosaurs. But to me, receiving a beautifully penned letter from a loved one carries so much meaning. Take the time to write to someone you truly care for. Invest in fine, personalized stationery and an exquisitely designed fountain pen to create your beautiful notes.

~ **Dig in your garden.** Revel in the freshly tilled soil. Wriggle your toes deep in the damp, living earth. Reconnect with Mother Nature. And don't forget to plant the seeds for super summer salads.

~ **Create a spiritual oasis.** I feel closer to God when I'm in my flower and herb garden than when I'm in a building. If space is limited or gardening is not your passion, create a private, serene space on your deck, in your bedroom, or in a corner of your living room. Decorate your personal sanctuary to reflect who you really are deep within. Perfume the area with frankincense (*Boswellia sacra*) essential oil. It has been used as an adjunct to prayer and meditation for centuries. If you don't have a diffuser, simply place the drops on a tissue and inhale deeply every few minutes. Frankincense helps balance mood swings and calm anxiety.

～ **Buy the best mattress and finest set of sheets you can possibly afford.** There's no substitute for sound, comfortable, luxuriant sleep.

Life is to be cherished and celebrated. Though food is essential to our physical well-being, our souls and spirits must be cared for and nourished, too — through the warmth and wonders of human connection, compassion, fellowship, intimacy, and our very presence on this provident earth. Always give freely of yourself, care about yourself and others, care for your planet, and welcome the blessings of life and love.

Let no one ever come to you without leaving better and happier.

—MOTHER TERESA

6

Become
Mentally Fit

A healthy attitude, daily exercise, stress management, and mental gymnastics: These are the major ingredients for a lifetime of mental fitness. Just what is mental fitness? Being mentally fit means having a sharp memory, a creative mind, a positive attitude, and an optimistic outlook on life. A healthy state of mind resists hopelessness, negativity, blame, despair, resentment, worry, ungratefulness, and anxiety.

The phrase *mental health and fitness* means something different to everyone. Being mentally fit goes hand in hand with a fit body; a satisfying, stimulating, and nurturing mental environment; personal and social evolution; and spiritual fulfillment. The mind and body do not function independently; rather, they are intimately linked, the health of one dependent on the health of the other.

Your Attitude Matters

Indeed it does! A good attitude is a valuable ingredient in a quality life. What is a healthy mental attitude? It is a positive outlook on life where there is abundant love, hope, graciousness, peace, joy, and gratefulness. These emotions enhance our inner being and our outward appearance.

To illustrate how attitude matters in relation to your health and well-being, I would be remiss not to mention Norman Cousins, author of *Anatomy of an Illness as Perceived by the Patient*, who had been diagnosed with a painful immunological disorder that began destroying the collagen in his tissues. "Incurable," he was told by his doctors. But during his illness, he watched lots of comedy films and videos, which helped him maintain a positive attitude in an otherwise depressing period of his life. Mr. Cousins referred to laughter as "inner jogging," a way to reduce tension, heighten awareness, and release pain-killing endorphins. Daily laughter and exposure to humorous situations promotes the flow of positive energy throughout the brain, boosting immune-system functioning and reducing stress. Humor heals.

Conversely, anger, worry, ungratefulness, sadness, negative thoughts, resentment, and feelings of inadequacy can actually depress the immune system, leading to more serious problems — such as chemical and hormonal imbalances, increased levels of pain, substance abuse, violence, and suicide.

Minds are like parachutes. They only function when they are open.

—Sir James Dewar

Ingredients for a Healthy Mental Attitude

Strive to fill your mind with uplifting thoughts and your days with feel-good activities. Such an approach leaves little room for negative influences, and your level of joy and quality of life will improve — guaranteed!

~ **Have faith.** Studies have shown that regular followers of a religious faith and those who believe in the power of prayer tend to have a more positive outlook on life, heal faster from illness, lead longer lives, and have lower blood pressure and less frequent bouts of depression. Religious folk regularly commune for worship and fellowship, forming strong bonds with like-minded people while strengthening their own family bonds.

～ **Give and receive affection with joy and gusto!** I believe that the loving energy you give to the universe will come back to you threefold. You are not the center of the universe; if you are in need of positive attention, affection, and appreciation, you must give it first. Giving affection simply means offering words of praise to people you feel deserve it, shaking hands with everyone you meet, greeting others with a friendly smile and pleasant word, lending an ear to someone who needs it, or helping a needy neighbor or friend when the chips are down. Don't expect to get affection in return all the time. What you will get for your efforts, though, is a sense of well-being and an inner peace. When you spread joy, joy returns.

～ **Keep happily busy and have many interests and hobbies.** A very busy person never has time to brood or be unhappy.

～ **Make the best of all circumstances.** None of us has everything we could possibly need and want; we all share some degree of sorrow and longing. No matter your situation, focus your thoughts and energies on the best possible things for yourself and your family.

Embrace Vitality and Nurture Health

Elizabeth Somer, M.A., R.D., author of *Age-Proof Your Body: Your Complete Guide to Lifelong Vitality,* recognizes the importance of holistic health. She says,

> The link between vitality and health is a win-win relationship. Embracing vitality boosts energy, helps maintain health, and reduces the risk of disease and premature aging. In turn, a healthier body encourages positive thinking and fuels vitality. Nurturing both works in your favor for health, happiness, and longevity.

Strive daily to embrace vitality and to nurture your health!

~ **Have purpose.** A strong sense of purpose in life is a must if you are to maintain a positive attitude. You are on this earth for a reason. Discover your passion and pursue it. Make your dream your work, and work your dream.

~ **Strive for excellence.** When you give your best daily, you will feel good about yourself. If you compromise your standards, you undermine your self-esteem.

~ **Exercise daily.** Daily exercise has a positive effect on negative stressors. Exercise, like laughter, produces relaxing, mood-enhancing endorphins that help you to better deal with whatever comes your way.

~ **Begin every day with affirmations.** Repeat each of the following sentences 3 times while standing in front of a mirror; say them with authority:

"I will have a fantastic day."

"Today is a blessing."

"I am getting better and wiser every day."

Feeling Depressed?

Everyone feels down in the dumps from time to time. It's a natural part of life. But if you find yourself unable to snap out of that feeling within a reasonable period, then it may be time to seek professional help.

Depression is an illness defined as a disturbance in an individual's emotions or moods, lasting every day for a period of 2 weeks or more, or a consistent feeling of

Don't borrow trouble. Imaginary things are harder to bear than actual ones.

—ROBERT LOUIS STEVENSON

being down for no apparent reason, thus preventing the successful living of normal day-to-day life. A stressful event — such as a death in the family, act of violence, physical accident, financial difficulty, or divorce — can trigger symptoms of depression, as well.

When considering a diagnosis of depression, the following are some of the symptoms a doctor will look for:

- Insomnia or disturbed sleep
- Fatigue and loss of energy
- Loss of interest in previously pleasurable activities and hobbies
- Suicidal or morbid thoughts or actions
- Feelings of low self-esteem, worthlessness, excessive guilt, lack of confidence
- Change in weight or appetite
- Consistently depressed mood
- Difficulty concentrating or decreased clarity of thought
- Avoidance of responsibility for fear of failure

Where can you go for help? Often the best place to start is your local Mental Health Association. (Check the Yellow

Pages for a listing.) Other helpful resources might include a family physician, family service agency, clergyperson, school counselor, psychiatric hospital, crisis center, reiki practitioner, psychologist, on-line chat room, hot line, marriage and family counselor, clinical social worker, nurse psychotherapist, or emergency room.

To rid yourself of that down-in-the-dumps feeling, many practitioners of holis-

Ode to Joy

In her book, *Body & Soul: Your Guide to Health, Happiness, and Total Well-Being,* Gail Harris inspires us to find joy everywhere: Like many things that are worthwhile, consciously adding happiness to our lives doesn't come without effort. Sometimes a sunset is so breathtakingly glorious, we can't help but notice; other times, the sinking sun spreads the merest blush of pink across a darkening sky. Either way, appreciating the wonder of the daily celestial light show begins with

tic medicine recommend first trying these suggestions: 30 minutes of *daily* vigorous exercise, standardized extract of St.-John's-wort (follow label directions), increased consumption of foods rich in omega-3 fatty acids (such as sardines and salmon, flaxseeds and oil, walnuts, and brazil nuts), vitamin B complex supplements, meditation, breathing exercises, and yoga.

I think, therefore I am.

—RENÉ DESCARTES

remembering to open our eyes. If joy is the end result of appreciation, appreciation comes from paying attention.

The best news is that whoever we are, wherever we live, whatever the state of our bank account, making the effort to connect with something larger than ourselves isn't so hard. You can start by going outside, taking a few deep breaths and looking up. It can be pretty dazzling, that sky. And it's there for us, all the time.

Your Environment and Your Mood

The connection between your home, work, and family environments and the state of your mind is widely accepted. The ancient Chinese science and art of feng shui, a 3,000-year-old environmental philosophy, is a practical way to improve many aspects of your life while balancing your environment.

In his book *Feng Shui Tips for a Better Life*, David Daniel Kennedy says, "Feng Shui is the art of using arrangement and placement to improve your life. It is a way of manipulating environmental factors to enhance the life energy of the environment and improve your destiny. Life energy, known as *chi* to the Chinese, is the basic force that animates all living things. Your own flow of chi will improve and strengthen as you apply Feng Shui principles to your life."

Your physical surroundings definitely have a significant impact on your moods. Next time you enter a cluttered room, whether it's in your home or office, take note of any physical sensations you experience. A room filled with too much stuff —

Since hate poisons the soul, don't cherish enmities and grudges.

—ROBERT LOUIS STEVENSON

too many objects, even if they are valuable artifacts — occupies too much "calming space" and can result in internal chaos.

Someone once told me that your home and workspaces mirror your internal condition — that your surroundings are a reflection of the emotional peace or turmoil you are currently experiencing in your life. I agree with this statement. Visual stimuli, whether good or bad, have a powerful impact on your mood.

The following are some suggestions for improving positive energy flow, both internally and externally, and for instilling harmony in your daily life:

∿ **Use simple, functional, aesthetically pleasing furnishings.** Too much of a good thing makes your rooms appear smaller and less warm. A room that appears crowded may simply need some tidying up or furniture rearrangement in order to provide a sense of expansiveness.

∿ **Organize.** Get rid of the stacks of magazines and piles of junk mail that you've been meaning to get to but haven't. Organize and file important items and toss out the rest.

~ **Don't procrastinate.** Either get the job done or just say no! Prioritize your daily schedule and keep it logged in one central place. A handy dated organizer or a computer notebook will work wonders for life simplification.

~ **Tidy up.** Keep every room at home or in the office as clean as possible. Dirt is distracting.

~ **Live and work in a well-lighted place.** The bedroom is the exception. Light lifts your mood and makes all rooms appear larger and brighter.

~ **Live with plants.** Plants are peace-givers. Place natural plants in all your surroundings to freshen the air, relax the eyes, and soothe a busy mind. If your budget is tight and you've only got a few pieces of furniture to fill a room, plants make the perfect, inexpensive furniture replacement.

Stay Mentally Sharp for Life

"Use dependent plasticity"; this is a neurological phrase for "use it or lose it." Scientists have long speculated that we are using only 10 percent of our brain capacity, leaving 90 percent of potential untapped. But what if you could access, cultivate, or unleash this vast creative energy?

In the daily practice of exercising your brain past its current limits, attempting to reach beyond the obvious solutions to a problem, new and permanent neural pathways in the brain will be created. Exercising the brain is believed to stimulate peak functioning. As you age, it is important to keep your mind active and not become a mental couch potato. Remaining mentally sharp is a key to aging well.

The best prescription is knowledge.

—Dr. C. Everett Koop

Scentual Therapy for the Mind

Essential oils of lemon, sage, peppermint, basil, nutmeg, sweet orange, ginger, and tangerine can help optimize mental performance, increase concentration, and clarify the mind. Essential oils of bergamot, lavender, myrrh, petitgrain, neroli, and ylang ylang can aid in balancing and centering your mood and emotions and promote happiness.

In order to forge ahead into uncharted mental territory and expand your thought processes you need to stimulate, challenge, and stretch your mind daily to keep it resilient, creative, and flexible. By challenging your brain to create new neural pathways you begin to open the untapped 90 percent of your brain. Additionally, this helps keep your memory and intelligence functioning at high levels.

Mental Gymnastics

Most of us grew up attending schools where the educational agenda was primarily to target the left side of the brain by requiring logical and rational studies (which used structured, sequential thought). Subjects such as reading, writing, mathematics, spelling, foreign language studies, and focused recreation (in which students work on jigsaw and crossword puzzles) filled this bill. Anything that makes you use logic, rationale, reason, and structured, sequential thought will engage the left side of your brain.

The right side of the brain is what many consider the "artsy" side. To stimulate this more creative part of your mind become involved with art, sports, and music and spatially oriented forms of learning and pattern recognition. You might want to learn more about landscape design, interior design, home building, pottery, sculpture, painting, weaving, sewing, or drawing. Dance lessons, yoga, t'ai chi, qi gong, reiki classes, and cosmetology studies also fall into this category. Right-brain learning nurtures the development of intuition and the ability to facilitate insight.

The best mental workouts involve stimulating the right and left sides of your brain. To accelerate your thinking, try doing things with the opposite hand. Write, dial the phone, brush your hair and teeth, apply your moisturizer, use the calculator, or move the computer mouse with your "lazy" hand. This teaches the nondominant side of your brain to develop coordination.

Challenge your brain by taking a break from routine. Drive a different route to work, take the kids to school instead of sending them out on the bus, wake up an hour earlier and meditate or take a walk, or rearrange your normal weekly activities.

The key to keeping the brain healthy for a lifetime is to exercise it on a daily basis. It's just like a muscle — it needs to work out in order to stay fit and functional.

The Thinking-Woman's Tea

Spur your creativity and mental awareness with this delicious herbal tea blend. The first two ingredients contain memory-enhancing and mind-stimulating compounds traditionally used to boost thinking power. All herbs in this recipe are in dried form.

> 6 teaspoons ginkgo leaves
>   (*Ginkgo biloba*)
> 3 teaspoons gotu kola leaves
>   (*Centella asiatica*)
> 3 teaspoons chamomile flowers
>   (*Matricaria recutita*)
> 2 teaspoons St.-John's-wort leaves
>   and flowers (*Hypericum perforatum*)
> 2 teaspoons lemon balm
>   (*Melissa officinalis*)
> 2 teaspoons peppermint
>   (*Mentha piperita*)
>   a pinch stevia extract powder
>   (*Stevia rebaudiana*)

1. In a medium-sized bowl, combine herbs.
2. For a large mug of tea, bring 1½ cups of purified water to a boil, then remove from heat. Add 2 teaspoons of the herbs, cover, and steep for 10 to 15 minutes.
3. Strain. Pour the tea into your favorite mug, adding a squeeze of lemon or orange to enhance flavor if desired. Enjoy hot or iced. One serving per day is recommended. Store leftover dried blend in an airtight, labeled tin, plastic tub, or plastic zipper bag. It will keep for up to 6 months in a cool, dark, dry place.

Yield: Approximately 9 large mugs of tea

There is no wealth but life.

—JOHN RUSKIN

Recommended Reading

Austin, John. "We Are Family." *Spirit of Change,* July/August 2000.

Batmanghelidj, Fereydoon. *Your Body's Many Cries for Water.* Falls Church, VA: Global Health Solutions, 1997.

Brody, Jane E. *Good Food Book — Living the High-Carbohydrate Way.* New York: Norton, 1985.

Cabot, Sandra, M.D. *The Liver Cleansing Diet: Love Your Liver and Live Longer.* Scottsdale, AZ: S.C.B. International, 1996.

Colbin, Annemarie. *The Book of Whole Meals.* New York: Ballantine, 1983.

Cousins, Norman. *Anatomy of an Illness as Perceived by the Patient.* New York: Bantam Doubleday Dell, 1991.

Gillanders, Ann. *The Joy of Reflexology: Healing Techniques for the Hands & Feet to Reduce Stress & Reclaim Health.* Boston: Little, Brown, 1996.

Gray, Robert. *The Colon Health Handbook.* Reno, NV: Emerald Publishing, 1995.

Harris, Gail. *Body & Soul: Your Guide to Health, Happiness, and Total Well-Being*. New York: Kensington Publishing, 1999.

Jones, Susan Smith. *Choose Radiant Health & Happiness*. Berkeley, CA: Celestial Arts, 1998.

Kabat-Zinn, Jon. *Wherever You Go, There You Are*. New York: Hyperion, 1994.

Kennedy, David Daniel. *Feng Shui Tips for a Better Life*. Pownal, VT: Storey Books, 1998.

Lawless, Julia. *The Illustrated Encyclopedia of Essential Oils: The Complete Guide to the Use of Oils in Aromatherapy and Herbalism*. Rockport, MA: Element Books, 1995.

Maddern, Jan. *Yoga Builds Bones: Easy Gentle Stretches That Prevent Osteoporosis*. Boston, MA: Element Books, 2000.

Malkmus, Rhonda J. *Recipes for Life from God's Garden*. Shelby, NC: Hallelujah Acres Publishing, 1998.

Marks, Linda. "The Village People Diet." *Spirit of Change* September/October 2000.

Maslow, Abraham H. *Toward a Psychology of Being,* 3rd ed. Richard Lowry, ed. New York: Wiley, 1998.

McDougall, John A., and Mary A. McDougall. *The McDougall Plan.* Piscataway, NJ: New Century Publishers, 1983.

Moran, Victoria. *Creating a Charmed Life: Sensible, Spiritual Secrets Every Busy Woman Should Know.* New York: HarperCollins, 1999.

Oliver, Joan Duncan. *Contemplative Living.* New York: Dell Publishing, 2000.

Ollsin, Don. *Herbal Healing Journey.* Victoria, BC: Aquiline Communications, 1998.

Page, Linda Rector, N.D., Ph.D. *How to Be Your Own Herbal Pharmacist: Herbal Traditions, Expert Formulations.* Carmel Valley, CA: Healthy Healing Publications, 1991.

Pitchford, Paul. *Healing with Whole Foods: Oriental Traditions and Modern Nutrition.* Berkeley, CA: North Atlantic Books, 1993.

Raichur, Pratima. *Absolute Beauty: Radiant Skin and Inner Harmony Through the Ancient Secrets of Ayurveda.* New York: HarperCollins, 1997.

Rechelbacher, Horst. *Aveda Rituals: A Daily Guide to Natural Health and Beauty.* New York: Henry Holt and Co., 1999.

———. *Rejuvenation: A Wellness Guide for Women and Men*. Rochester, VT: Healing Arts Press, 1987.

Schulze, Richard. *Get Well!* May 2000.

Somer, Elizabeth, M.A., R.D. *Age-Proof Your Body: Your Complete Guide to Lifelong Vitality*. New York: William Morrow, 1998.

Walton, Izaac, and Charles Cotton. *The Compleat Angler: Or the Contemplative Man's Recreation,* reprint edition. New York: Random House, 1998.

Weil, Andrew. *Eating Well for Optimum Health*. New York: Knopf, 2000.

Weinberg, Norma Pasekoff. *Natural Hand Care*. Pownal, VT: Storey Books, 1998.

Wildish, Paul. *The Book Of Ch'i*. Boston, MA: Tuttle Publishing, 2000.

Worwood, Valerie Ann. *The Complete Book of Essential Oils and Aromatherapy*. San Rafael, CA: New World Library, 1991.

Resources

Herbs, Natural Products, Sunscreen

A-Cute Derm
7800 Bissonnet Street,
  Building 455
Houston, TX 77074-5423
800-922-2883
Web site: www.a-cutederm.com
Manufacturer of PRO-TECT broad-spectrum sunscreens. Free catalog and fascinating sun protection information.

**The American Botanical
  Pharmacy**
P.O. Box 9699
Marina Del Rey, CA 90295
800-437-2362
Organically grown and wild-harvested herbal preparations. Highly recommended! Free catalog.

Aubrey Organics
4419 North Manhattan Avenue
Tampa, FL 33614
800-282-7394
Web site: www.aubrey-organics.com
Manufacturer of 100% natural skin, hair, and body care products. Free catalog.

Aura Cacia
P.O. Box 311
Norway, IA 52318
800-437-3301
Web site: www.frontiercoop.com
Source for natural essential oils and related items. Free catalog.

Frontier Cooperative Herbs
3021 78th Street
Norway, IA 52318
800-786-1388
Web site: www.frontierherb.com
Supplier of organic and wildcrafted bulk herbs and herbal products. Free catalog.

Jean's Greens
Herbal Tea Works & Herbal
  Essentials
119 Sulphur Spring Road
Norway, New York 13416
888-845-TEAS (8327)
Fax 315-845-6501
Web site: www.jeansgreens.com
E-mail: jean@jeansgreens.com
This shop carries just about everything you'll need for the skin-care products in this book. Reasonable prices, friendly service. Free catalog.

Kathleen's Herbs
P.O. Box 551
Hyannisport, MA 02647
508-790-1690
A wellness and healing center offering aromatherapy, herbs, reiki sessions, herbal oils, lotions, soaps, skin care, classes and demonstrations, and spiritual healing.

Mountain Rose Herbs
20818 High Street
North San Juan, CA 95960
800-879-3337
Fax 510-217-4012
Web site: www.mountainrose
    herbs.com
Organically grown herbs, herb seeds, base oils, essential oils, bottles, jars, hair- and skin-care products, tinctures, salves, and teas. Free catalog.

Original Swiss Aromatics
P.O. Box 6842
San Rafael, CA 94903
415-459-3998
Fax 415-479-0614
Web site: www.pacificinstituteof
    aromatherapy.com
Superior quality "genuine and authentic" (ge³a) and vintage essential oils. They specialize in providing absolutely genuine, and frequently organic, essential oils from farmers and distillers. Free catalog.

**September's Sun Herbal Soap
    & Skin Care Company**
Stephanie Tourles, owner
P.O. Box 772
West Hyannisport, MA 02672
508-862-9955
Fax 508-778-9262
E-mail: stourles@mediaone.net
Handmade herbal goat milk soaps, skin-care products formulated by a licensed esthetician and aromatherapist, and personally signed herb books. Send SASE for free product brochure.

Simplers Botanical Co.
P.O. Box 2534
Sebastopol, CA 95473
800-652-7646
Fax 707-887-7570
Web site: www.simplers.com
Pharmaceutical-grade essential oils, herbal oil infusions, real perfume oils, and aromatic hydrosols. Excellent essential oils for the aromatherapist or skin-care professional. Free catalog.

American Academy of Dermatology
930 North Meacham Road
Schaumburg, IL 60173
888-462-DERM (3376)
Web site: www.aad.org
Excellent source for physician referrals and free brochures on skin health and disorders. Very educational!

American Heart Association
National Center
7272 Greenville Avenue
Dallas, TX 75231
Women's Health Information line: 888-MY-HEART (694-3278)
Web site: www.americanheart.org
Free heart health brochures.

American Institute of Stress
124 Park Avenue
Yonkers, NY 10703
914-963-1200
Fax 914-965-6267
Web site: www.stress.org
E-mail: stress124@earthlink.net
Free fascinating information on the benefits of sleep and sleep-deficit disorders.

International Institute of Reflexology
5650 First Avenue North
St. Petersburg, FL 33733
727-343-4811
Web site: www.reflexology-USA.net
Free training seminar information and certified reflexologist referrals.

National Institute on Aging
Building 31, Room 5C27
31 Center Drive / MSC 2292
Bethesda, MD 20892
301-496-1752
Web site: www.nih.gov/nia
Free brochures and information on aging issues.

National Mental Health Association
1021 Prince Street
Alexandria, VA 22314-2971
800-969-NMHA
Web site: www.nmha.org
E-mail: infoctr@nmha.org
Free fact sheets available on variety of mental-health topics.

The Skin Cancer Foundation
P.O. Box 561
New York, NY 10156
800-SKIN-490
Web site: www.skincancer.org
E-mail: info@skincancer.org
Free information on skin cancer.

Index

Other Storey Titles You Will Enjoy

50 Simple Ways to Pamper Yourself by Stephanie Tourles. With recipes, tips, and techniques for giving your body and mind the care they deserve, this book helps you relieve stress, promote relaxation, and beautify every part of your body. 144 pages. Paperback. ISBN 1-58017-210-5.

The Herbal Body Book by Stephanie Tourles. Discover how to transform common herbs, fruits, and grains into safe, economical, and natural personal-care items. Includes more than 100 recipes for facial scrubs, shampoos, lip balms, moisturizers, and much more. 128 pages. Paperback. ISBN 0-88266-880-3.

Herbs for Reducing Stress and Anxiety by Rosemary Gladstar. One of America's foremost herbalists provides concise, simple, and practical information for using herbs to relieve stress and anxiety. 96 pages. Paperback. ISBN 1-58017-155-9.

Natural Foot Care by Stephanie Tourles. From easy-to-make recipes for creams, lotions, and ointments to foot massage techniques, this book offers dozens of natural ways to care for feet. 192 pages. Paperback. ISBN 1-58017-054-4.

7 Simple Steps to Unclutter Your Life by Donna Smallin. For readers who yearn for more balance in their lives, this book offers hundreds of tips and ideas for enhancing physical, emotional, and spiritual well-being while creating a simpler, less stressful lifestyle. 176 pages. Paperback. ISBN 1-58017-237-7.

365 Ways to Energize Mind, Body & Soul by Stephanie Tourles. This unique idea-a-day book delivers energizing recipes, practical and easy-to-implement ideas, and sound, friendly advice that will help readers feel healthy, happy, and fully alive. 384 pages. Paperback. ISBN 1-58017-331-4.

365 Ways to Relax Mind, Body & Soul by Barbara L. Heller. From simple, uplifting thoughts to soothing exercises to relaxing foods and diet advice, this book offers effective ways to beat stress and promote relaxation in a fun, idea-a-day format. 384 pages. Paperback. ISBN 1-58017-332-2.

These books and other Storey books are available at your bookstore, farm store, garden center, or directly from Storey Books, Schoolhouse Road, Pownal, Vermont 05261, or by calling 1-800-441-5700. Or visit our Web site at www.storeybooks.com